Dr. Kidd's Guide to

Herbal Cat Care

Randy Kidd, D.V.M., Ph.D.

STOREY BOOKS

Schoolhouse Road
Pownal, Vermont 05261

*The mission of Storey Communications is to serve our customers
by publishing practical information that encourages personal
independence in harmony with the environment.*

Edited by Deborah Burns, Robin Catalano, and Karen Levy
Cover design by Meredith Maker
Cover photograph of cat by Artville; cover photograph of garden by Giles
    Prett/SCI
Back cover illustration and animal illustrations by Rick Daskam
Herbal illustrations by Bobbi Angell, Kathy Bray, Sarah Brill, Beverly Duncan,
    Brigita Fuhrmann, Regina Hughes, Charles Joslin, Alison Kolesar, Susan
    Berry Langsten, and Doug Paisley
Text design by Susan Bernier
Text production by Jennifer Jepson Smith and Deborah Daly
Indexed by Susan Olason

Printed in the United States by Versa Press
10 9 8 7 6 5 4 3 2 1

Library of Congress Cataloging-in-Publication Data

Kidd, Randy, 1942-
    [Guide to herbal cat care]
    Dr. Kidd's guide to herbal cat care/Randy Kidd.
        p. cm
    ISBN 1-58017-188-5 (pbk. : alk. paper)
        1. Cats—Diseases—Alternative treatment. 2. Herbs—Therapeutic use.
        3. Herbals. 4. Holistic veterinary medicine. I. Title: Guide to herbal cat
        care. II. Title.
SF985 .K54 2000
636.8'08955—dc21   00-061873

Contents

Acknowledgments

Writers draw strength and inspiration from many sources, and I'd like to acknowledge three statements of belief that have formed the foundation of my approach to holistic veterinary medicine:

"In the beginning of all things, wisdom and knowledge were with the animals; for Tirawa, the One Above, did not speak directly to man. He sent the animals to tell man that he showed himself through the beasts, and that from them, and from the stars and the sun and the moon, man should learn."
    Chief Latakots-Lesa, Pawnee Tribe

"We believe that the domestic animals were sent here to accept the diseases of humans . . . and to show them how to heal these diseases."
    Tis Mal Crow, Native American "Root Doctor"

"If there were no plants we would not be here. We breathe in what they breathe out. That is how we learn from them."
    Keetoowah, Cherokee Teacher

I would also like to thank my hundreds of four-legged patients for their role as my teachers. My wife Sue is my strength, my way of staying rooted to the wellness that comes from our Earth Mother. Finally, I'd like to thank the folks at Storey Books for their editorial input and for having the faith that this book will help your pet's health, naturally.

part 1

Introducing Herbs

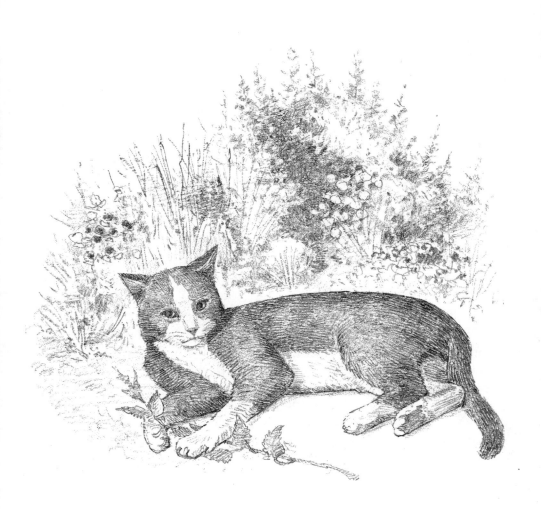

Introduction to Herbalism

Herbs have been an integral part of humankind's diet and pharmacy since we began roaming the earth. The ancient Sumerians left written evidence of medicinal uses for plants such as laurel, caraway, and thyme some five thousand years ago. But long before the written word, caveman cultures left evidence of herbal use in their coprolites, or fossilized excrement. Herbalists have practiced their trade since the time of recorded history and in all parts of the world. Many herbs are mentioned in the Bible.

Typically, the plants of yore were used in unity with nature; their medicinal uses were based on humans' intuitive feel for their application along with observed results. Herbal use was often combined with practices such as shamanism, bleeding, fumigation, poulticing, rubbing, and urtication. In addition, most cultures combined a ritualistic approach to planting and harvesting and the collection of wild species.

Today, our culture so relies on Western medicines that we have lost perspective on herbs. But herbs are used by more people worldwide than any other medicine. You probably don't have to go very far back in your own family history (perhaps to your grandmother or great-aunt) to discover an herbalist, someone who used the local "weeds" to cure all sorts of ailments.

Despite all this herbal history and lore, folks sometimes seem reluctant to use herbal medicines to help their pets. Concerned animal lovers have questions: Are the herbs safe to use? Which ones can I use for my cat? When should I use herbs, and are they ever more appropriate than the drugs of Western medicine? Should I use capsules, teas, tinctures, or topical herbs? How do I dose these treatments? And finally, are herbal medicines effective?

This book is designed to answer those questions. Herbs have been an integral part of my holistic practice for the past 10 years, and they have also been a part of my family's health care for several generations. Herbs are so safe and effective as helpers for other alternative medicines that I give almost every one of my patients an herbal prescription. And after years of use on hundreds of kitty patients — including my own cats — I have found the herbs so safe (when used correctly) that I am extremely comfortable prescribing them for all critters, even the most profoundly sick.

WHAT IS HOLISTIC MEDICINE?

I am a holistic veterinarian and have been one for about 10 years. I use a variety of "medicines" in my practice: herbs, acupuncture (Traditional Chinese Medicine), homeopathy, spinal and limb adjustments (chiropractic), nutrition and nutritional supplements, flower essences, shamanism, and more. Occasionally, I even resort to the Western or allopathic medicine I learned in veterinary school. I use what I think will be best for the patient at a particular time in his life cycle. And over the years I've found that, more often than not, the alternative medicines I choose *do* work.

Holistic medicine is much more than the "medicines" used. It is an approach to wellness that looks at the patient as a whole organism, an organism that is intimately connected to its natural environment and whose health is tied to the health and well-being of the other organisms (including humans) around it.

St.-John's-wort

How Does Holistic Medicine Work?

Holistic medicine assumes that a diseased part of the organism is merely an expression of the fact that a lack of balance exists somewhere within the body. When seeking a cure for any disease, a holistic practitioner tries to create a balance among all the body's organ systems.

To effect that cure, a holistic practitioner must be able to look at the patient from many different perspectives. Each of the medicines I use — herbal, homeopathic, Eastern, chiropractic, Western — has its own diagnostic and therapeutic methodology. And each of these methodologies is an independent system of its own, often complex and intricate in its approach and certainly highly refined by years of successful use by countless practitioners and patients.

Taking Responsibility for Health and the Planet

An additional aspect of holistic medicine that I feel is critical to the overall concept of "wholism" is that the medicine must be natural and must not deplete or pollute the environment.

Finally, and perhaps most important, I believe that holistic medicine — and especially the use of herbal remedies — is a prime way of empowering people to take charge of their pets' health . . . and their own.

When using herbal medicines, you are the specialist. As an herbalist you realize that foods (and especially herbs) are medicine; medicine is food. And you give your cat a boost with a daily dose of healthy herbs. Herbs are readily available over the counter for easy access. You don't need someone with a bunch of letters after his name to write a prescription just so you can use herbs; you can use herbs because you know they are safe and effective and because they work in a wide variety of situations, often affecting several organ systems at once. You don't need a zillion bucks' worth of diagnostic and treatment machinery to support your healing methods; the herbs are there for you because healing is their job. And, perhaps best of all, you can grow healthy herbs in your very own backyard.

My Beginnings as a Practicing Herbalist

While my family has made extensive use of herbs seemingly forever, my dog, Rufus, finally convinced me to use them in my practice. (Remember, like that of all my veterinary colleagues, my previous training was exclusively oriented toward Western medicine.)

Rufus: My First Case Study

Just about the time I began studying alternative medicines, Rufus, a totally lovable golden retriever with the usual complement of three brain cells, got a "hot spot" on his forearm. Hot spots are skin irritations of unknown cause that usually begin as small, itchy areas that the animal may lick and bite until the spots are raw and bleeding. In Western medicine hot spots are commonly treated by applying cortisone ointment, an anti-inflammatory.

I gave Rufus the best of Western medicine, slathering on the cortisone ointment. His hot spot went away almost immediately. But it returned in a few months — redder, angrier, and itchier. So I went to the bigger "guns" of Western medicine: oral cortisone pills, given in addition to the topical ointment.

The hot spot disappeared, this time after three or four days . . . only to return again in a few months. The spot was redder yet, much larger, and, according to Rufus, so itchy it was nearly impossible to bear. I gave him another dose of cortisone, this time in ointment, injectable, and follow-up pill form.

The hot spot again disappeared, this time after a week or so. But in a few weeks it came back with a vengeance, and Rufus let us know he was miserable, day and night. Well, you get the picture. Western medicines in general, and cortisone products in particular, typically work by palliating diseases — making patients feel better for short periods of time without really curing them.

Calendula

Finding Success with Herbs

By now deep into my alternative medicine studies, I decided to apply what I'd learned to Rufus. (Much like the shoemaker's daughter who never has shoes, most veterinarians' pets are the last to get treated.) From the few herbal books I had at the time, I learned that calendula is a good herb for healing reddened, raw skin lesions. Sue, my wife, had some calendula growing in the garden, so we picked it, steeped it into a mild tea, and spritzed it on Rufus's ever-growing hot spot.

"Ahhh." I could almost hear Rufus's sigh of relief as he settled in, quit scratching, and relaxed for the first time in days. In a few hours the itch reccurred, so we applied another spritz. Immediate relief. After four or five treatments throughout that first day, Rufus experienced no itching, and he had a good night's sleep for the first time in weeks. Then, amazingly, the very next morning I could see evidence of wound healing around the edges of the hot spot — nice white, clean tissue growth.

Well, after a few days of herbal spritzing, Rufus's hot spot completely disappeared, and it has never returned. I was really happy for Rufus (and for us, since we could now sleep), but I wondered why I hadn't learned about calendula or any of the other herbs in veterinary school. But that's another story.

After watching Rufus's results, I was hooked. I began using herbs extensively from that day on, recommending them for all my patients.

HOW TO USE THIS BOOK

Dr. Kidd's Guide to Herbal Cat Care is designed to make it easy for you to begin using herbs on your kitty right away. Please read the first section before you jump into the chapters on organ systems and the herbal repertory.

Chapters 4 and 5 are designed to help you understand the how-tos of herbal use. But there's nothing difficult about it. Herbal medicine is not rocket science. I am a veterinarian and an herbalist who thinks of herbal medicine as the most empowering of the alternative medicines because it is meant to be used by everyone — including your cat. *You* can choose to create a healthy internal and external environment by growing and feeding herbs to your animals. *You* can choose to use herbs because they are safe and effective. And, as you use herbs, *you* can learn about your own environment (and especially your own backyard environment) and the place herbs have in it.

Start using herbs today. Sprinkle a sample of a tonic herb atop Mittens's food. If she doesn't like that tonic, try another. Keep trying until you find the herbs she likes. Make a light herbal tea and pour it over her food, or try adding some to her water.

To keep your cat healthy, use herbs on a daily basis. Should the unfortunate occasion ever occur, you'll have much better luck getting a sick kitty to agree to herbal medicines if she has been acclimated to them over the years.

Then, if your cat ever does come down with the "sicks," all you need is a diagnosis from your "regular" veterinarian that tells you which organ system is affected or which special problem your cat has. With the diagnosis in hand, go to the chapter that lists the herbs for that organ system, and use them as directed. It couldn't be simpler.

Now there is a minor rub to all of this: Whenever you choose to use herbal medicine (or any other alternative medicine, for that matter), you most likely won't get much help (or *any* help) from your conventional veterinarian. Such vets are simply not trained in holistic health care. But holistic veterinarians are now located in all parts of North America (see Resources), and many of them are available for either office or phone consultations. In any emergency, of course, you should contact your regular vet or local emergency veterinary clinic.

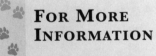

FOR MORE INFORMATION

For those of you who want to continue your herbal studies, or for those who want to have some more fun with herbs, check out my two Web sites: www.HookedOnHerbs.com and www.HonoringThe Animals.com.

10 Steps to Holistic Medicine for Cats

As I've mentioned, holistic medicine is much more than any one medicine. So, early on in my holistic practice, I developed a protocol that has helped me think in terms of wholism — an integrated approach to creating whole-body-mind-heart-spirit health for Pet (and for Pet's people). I know many holistic practitioners who refer to this holistic balance as body-mind-spirit (or body-mind-soul). But I separate the heart and spirit because I've always thought of the heart as an internally located organ *and* source of energy, while I see the spirit as more outwardly oriented — an unknown source that dramatically affects all internal organs. This heart-spirit split may be merely semantics, but it gives me the opportunity to describe and work with a cat's brave predator heart, or a cat that has a "broken heart" over the loss of a family member.

Interestingly, Traditional Chinese Medicine has a term, *shen,* which is identified as "spirit," or the substance unique to human life. Human consciousness indicates the presence of shen. Shen resides in the heart, along with what the Chinese view as the mind.

Finally, I see spirit and soul as the same. But this gets some holistic veterinarians in trouble with the folks who don't think animals have souls. In addition, my protocol has helped me see where the herbs fit (or at least where *I* think they fit) in an overall approach to wellness.

For my protocol I use a highly scientific model: one of those bathtub toys made for kids. (My idea for using the bathtub toy came as I watched one of our grandkids splash in the tub. What could be more healthy than watching kids or pets have fun?) This protocol forces us to be aware of the holistic perspective of wellness. It also helps us apply the healing methods we ultimately select in proper sequence. And from its format, we can learn to think about *all* aspects of health in a logical, sequential manner.

Healer Cats

Some of my professional colleagues think I'm weird, but as a scientist I can't help but record some of my observations. One of the aspects of cats that I find the most fascinating is their apparent ability to take on the family role of the "healer cat." The healer cat is the family feline that is always hanging around whenever anyone is sick, always there to rub up against, purr for, and lie with the sick individual — whether it is a two-legged or four-legged patient.

Healer cats have the uncanny ability to know *who* is sick and *where* the sickness is in the individual's body. The cats typically lie on or near that spot, as if to absorb any negative energy. Clients tell me that their healer cats know when they have a stomachache, and the cat will sit on their belly while they are lying on the couch trying to recover. Others say that if they have a headache, the healer cat will lie next to their head until the ache goes away. I've had too many clients tell me these stories to allow me to ignore them.

I've also noticed that it is not always just one cat in the family that is a healer cat. And, interestingly, when a healer cat passes on, another family cat typically assumes the role.

HOW TO INTERPRET THE MODEL

My protocol is based on a direct connection with Mother Earth, creating a basis of holistic health that relies on living *naturally*. In addition, any holistic approach to health will create a natural balance of body, mind, heart, and spirit.

**DR. KIDD'S HOLISTIC PROTOCOL FOR HEALTH:
AS ONE WITH NATURE**

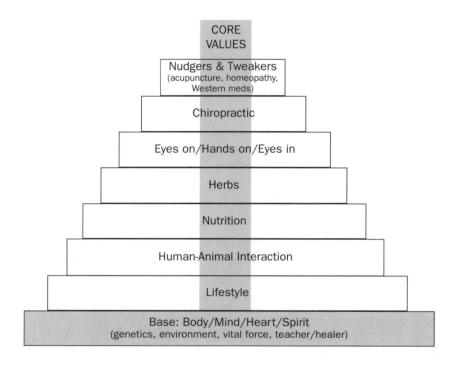

CORE
VALUES

Nudgers & Tweakers
(acupuncture, homeopathy,
Western meds)

Chiropractic

Eyes on/Hands on/Eyes in

Herbs

Nutrition

Human-Animal Interaction

Lifestyle

Base: Body/Mind/Heart/Spirit
(genetics, environment, vital force, teacher/healer)

The Foundation: As One with Nature

I think it helps to visualize my model as resting on a healthy Mother Earth, seeking natural ways to evaluate and perpetuate health. Then, envision an application of the protocol that always includes a natural way to balance all the aspects of body, mind, heart, and spirit. Finally, think in terms of the animal being able to heal itself, working with its own innate powers. This, then, is the first and perhaps most important step in the protocol: realizing that everything we do for ourselves and for our animals is based on the premise that we are all one with nature. The realization of this interconnectedness with nature will ultimately make us and our pets whole and healthy.

Just as you would begin with the base when building anything with structural integrity, you must establish a firm foundation for holistic health. Next, look closely at each of the rings, proceeding from the larger rings at the bottom to the smaller rings at the top. The larger the ring, the greater the emphasis required on that area of health.

Also, remember that as you proceed from the bottom to the top of the model, your ability to tweak the patient's vital force *(chi)* toward wellness is progressively stronger — as are your chances to harm the patient if the method used is not applied properly. This means that you should not use any of the potent medicines, including homeopathy, chiropractic, or acupuncture, *unless* you have the knowledge base that comes from adequate training in the method.

The Base

The base, or foundation, of my model is made up of several factors. All of these factors must be present for optimum health.

Genetics. The basis of any wellness program is a genetic foundation that produces immune-competent and socially adaptable animals. Unfortunately, many commercial breeding programs breed for a special look — a particular hair or eye color, for example, or a long snout. When animal breeds try to get one specific look, the genes necessary for a robust immune system, good behavior, mothering ability, or other important aspects of a whole and healthy animal often aren't passed on. In other words, the price we pay for "looks-specific" genetics may be generations of offspring that are not holistically sound.

Environment. All animals (including humans) have the right to live in a pollution-free, stress-free, toxin-free environment — an outer environment that allows the animal to meet its natural needs.

Vital force. For whole-body-mind-heart-spirit wellness, the vital force (or chi, or innate, or spirit, or orgone, or whatever else you might want to call it) must be able to grow to its capacity. I've found herbs, especially when used with the energetic medicines of homeopathy and acupuncture, to be vital in this area.

Animals as teachers and healers. The essence of our association with animals is to love and honor them as teachers — our very best models for natural, holistic health.

The Lower Rings

The rings sit atop the base of the model. Just as the base is composed of several factors, there are a variety of rings. Each ring corresponds to a different aspect of holistic health care.

Lifestyle. Every lifestyle choice a person makes has the potential to affect the overall health of her entire family of animals. Smoking, for example, not only harms the smoker but also damages her cat's lungs through secondary smoke. But when a family eats a wholesome, organic, balanced diet, the family cat has the added advantage of getting healthy table scraps. When the family engages the cat in a daily play session, all the players benefit from the exercise.

Human-animal interaction. All animals crave interaction with other living beings. Research shows that merely touching an animal lowers a person's heart rate. Human conversations even become quieter in the presence of animals. And simply watching animals — a fish in an aquarium is enough — calms the observers and lowers their blood pressure. Watch the animals, and it becomes clear that they

Regular interaction with your cat is integral to her general health and well-being.

also need the benefit of touch, from other animals and from their humans. The impressive part of human-animal interactions is that they work so well as a positive feedback system: The more we touch and rub and hug, the more each of us benefits. The healthier we become, the healthier our pets are, too.

Nutrition. The best food for all animals (again, including humans) is organic and natural. The worst is derived from diseased meat scraps, grains produced with heavy doses of herbicides and pesticides, highly cooked foods, and feed sources laden with artificial preservatives or flavorings. Provide the best quality nutrients available, and 90 percent of Pet's health problems will miraculously disappear. Remember: Herbs are also healthy foods.

The Middle Rings

Building on the base and lower rings, we can view the middle rings as important supplemental health care methods.

Herbs. Herbs can provide a full spectrum of impact on the vital force. Many of the herbs can be used as vitamins and immune-enhancing supplements, some are mild tonics or stimulants for numerous organ systems, and others are used as acute treatments. Although I've found some of the herbs to be extremely effective as therapeutic medicinals, as a general rule I consider them to be supportive for other health modalities. Typically the effects of herbs are very subtle, and it takes time (often 30 to 90 days) before we see positive results.

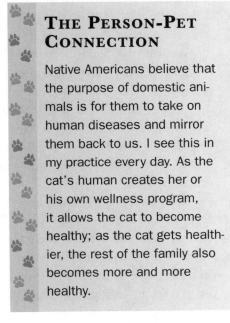

THE PERSON-PET CONNECTION

Native Americans believe that the purpose of domestic animals is for them to take on human diseases and mirror them back to us. I see this in my practice every day. As the cat's human creates her or his own wellness program, it allows the cat to become healthy; as the cat gets healthier, the rest of the family also becomes more and more healthy.

Hands on, Eyes on, Eyes in. A vital link from your heart to your cat's runs through your hands and through the positive images you produce of your cat's continuing health. Easy-to-learn massage techniques (hands on) will help transfer your innate healing powers to your cat, and the use of positive imagery (eyes in) will enhance any healthy method used for you or for the cat. Another key to a holistic health program is to properly evaluate your cat's ongoing condition. Good observational skills (eyes on) and the maintenance of a detailed journal are invaluable aids while helping Pet become and remain healthy.

Chiropractic. Many types of musculoskeletal pain or gait abnormalities can be eased with chiropractic care, and routine adjustments may be helpful for the athletic animal or human. In addition, a musculoskeletal system with a "kink" in it will not allow the vital force to flow freely. Often a simple chiropractic adjustment frees the animal's innate ability to balance and heal itself.

The Upper Rings: Nudgers and Tweakers

As you can see in the illustration on page 10, the top ring — what I call the nudgers and tweakers — is the smallest of the rings. While nudgers and tweakers have their place in health care, for long-term, in-depth holistic health, they are the least important of the 10 steps of the protocol.

Western medicine. Since it is the medicine most healing practitioners in the United States learn in school, Western (or allopathic) medicine is the kind of medicine that is practiced most predominantly in the United States. While all holistic practitioners are very aware of allopathic medicine's limitations, some applications have a place in any holistic practice. For example, allopathic medicine works very well when treating acute bacterial infections and traumatic injuries.

Acupuncture. Technically, acupuncture is only a portion of Traditional Chinese Medicine (TCM). True TCM also includes the use of Chinese herbs, lifestyle changes, chi mind/body exercises, and proper nutrition. Most U.S. practitioners, however, use acupuncture as the major part of TCM.

By selectively placing acupuncture needles along the naturally occurring meridians (lines of chi flow that the Chinese mapped out thousands of years ago) of an animal whose chi is not balanced, the practitioner achieves a healthy flow of energy that ultimately balances the animal's inner and outer wellness. Although TCM has been used for nearly all ailments in almost all species, it has proven to be especially helpful in animals (human and nonhuman) with painful musculoskeletal diseases.

Homeopathy. Homeopathy uses extremely diluted natural substances (from animal, vegetable, and mineral sources) that enable an animal's vital force to expand to its full capacity, thus eliminating the potential for impending diseases. The basis for homeopathy is that "like cures like," and healing remedies are selected according to the properties they have demonstrated in trials conducted on healthy people and animals. Homeopathic remedies have proven effective in all sorts of diseases, such as metabolic and musculoskeletal conditions.

Whole, organic foods are the foundation of a healthy diet.

Core Values

The central part of the model, the part that holds it all together, is what I call core values. Everyone has a set of core values he or she believes in implicitly. A person's spiritual beliefs are one example of a core value, and this value carries with it tremendous capacity for healing. No matter what your spiritual preference, prayer is a highly recommended — and proven effective — healing method for the entire family.

Wrapping It Up

So there you have the 10-Step Protocol I've found tremendously valuable for helping me decide the best holistic method I can use to effect long-term and in-depth healing. Everything is based on a natural approach; The entire protocol rests on Mother Earth, the basic premise of As One With Nature.

Nudgers and Tweakers

I consider all the powerful medicines I use — Western medicine, acupuncture, and homeopathy — as mere nudgers and tweakers because that's how I see them work clinically. Any of these medicines can nudge or tweak your cat into a healthier state of balance, at least temporarily.

However, for your cat's long-term wellness, I've found it is absolutely essential to establish a firm foundation of health (as per my holistic protocol). Otherwise, our "cures" are typically short-term and the disease returns — either in its original form or in another, often worse, chronic form of disease.

The major mistake of modern medicine, as I see it, is that it has flipped the protocol's pyramid and uses as its primary treatments the top, or smallest of the rings: the nudgers and tweakers. With the flip-flop, we have created a medicine without foundation, a medicine that has almost no structural integrity, a medicine that may work for the short term but does not create long-lasting health.

Using Herbs
for Health

From my perspective as a holistic practitioner, herbs offer the best of all worlds. Herbs have a full spectrum of activity, from mildly nutritional to powerfully medicinal. With this broad activity, herbal medicine gives us the opportunity to pick and choose the plants that will most likely help our patient's current condition.

Herbs are not drugs. For those of us with an allopathic background, this can be an extremely difficult concept to grasp. But if we are to use herbs successfully on our cats, it is absolutely essential that we understand this basic difference between drugs and herbs.

An herb is *not* one single bioactive chemical that a practitioner uses specifically to alter a biochemical process that has gone awry. Instead, each and every herb contains dozens of bioactive chemicals. As we'll see later, this potpourri of bioactive chemicals has its advantages and its drawbacks. Generally, herbs:

- **Are nutritional.** They add proteins, carbohydrates, vitamins, minerals, and other important nutrients (such as antioxidants) to the diet.
- **Add spice.** As well as being nutritional, and in many cases medicinal, culinary herbs add a spicy taste to foods. Spices not only enhance the taste of foods but also improve digestion by activating digestive juices and enzymes. Often just the odor of a spice will kick the digestive system into full gear.
- **Are tonic.** Many herbs have a tonic effect on the body, helping maintain the balance of the body's organ systems. A

tonic herb will either stimulate or relax its target organ systems, depending on what is needed. (See pages 19–20 for more information.)

- **Have specific medicinal uses.** Herbs used as medicine have a specific activity on one or several organ systems. In addition, they may have a specific activity, such as being effective against microorganisms. For instance, catnip is used to relax the nervous system, and it also has the ability to help clear up stomach upsets, such as colic, dyspepsia, and flatulence. Or herbs may be used to create a generalized physiological effect on the body — sweating, for example.
- **Can be contraindicated.** There are some herbs that should not be used during specific times of the life cycle, such as pregnancy. Other herbs are toxic enough that indiscriminate and prolonged use can lead to illness or even death. In addition, a few plants can be lethal, even in small, one-time, doses. Proper disease diagnosis and plant identification and dosage are absolutely necessary.

I think of secondary herbs as having activity associated with the organ system of concern, but not necessarily directly affecting it. For example, dandelion root acts as a diuretic, helping cleanse and nourish the urinary system. But I also often include it as a secondary herb for cardiac patients, because many animals with heart problems have a difficult time eliminating fluids and, thus, benefit from a diuretic herb.

CAUTION

Herbs can be beneficial, but if they are used incorrectly they may be toxic or even lethal. But the risk of adverse side effects and death is far less when using herbs than when using Western medicine's drugs. Now, admittedly, herbs are not without adverse reactions. But most of the herbal reactions seen are idiosyncratic, meaning they occur only in the rare individual who has a personal allergy to something in the herb.

It is estimated that ten thousand deaths a year are caused by allopathic drugs. Some experts even say this number is two or three times too low. If you added up all the deaths from herbal use, you *might* come up with one hundred over a 10-year period. You do the math.

Diagnosing and Prescribing

Correct diagnosis is essential in order to apply any medicine properly, and herbal medicine is no exception. However, each medical modality has its own specific diagnostics. Chinese medicine, for example, makes extensive use of tongue and pulse diagnosis. Classical homeopathy uses the totality of symptoms (without much regard to *why* the symptoms occur), while chiropractic uses joint flexibility and function as its primary diagnostic aids. Herbal medicine is no exception to this rule.

For herbal medicines, my primary interest is to determine which organ system is "out of whack" and needs to be returned to normal. Then, after I've determined the herbs that are specific for the affected organ system, I try to select herbs that will help other body

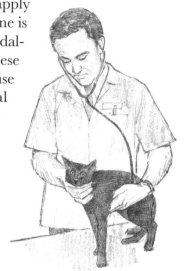

Always consult a qualified veterinarian before starting a treatment program.

systems that are also stressed by the cat's condition. In my practice, I follow a four-step process for diagnosing and prescribing.

Step 1: A Good Western Medicine Diagnosis

We need to know which of the cat's organ systems are compromised; we do not necessarily need to know the precise cause of the disease (though that can be helpful). Western medicine has excellent diagnostic tools for determining when an organ system is not normal: complete blood counts (CBCs), urinalysis, blood chemistries, X rays, magnetic resonance imaging (MRI), or ultrasound diagnosis may be indicated.

Let's say these tests indicate a dysfunctional urinary tract. In that case you would go to chapter 21 and select from the herbs that are listed as primary for the urinary system.

Step 2: Look for Outside Factors

Is the condition infectious or noninfectious? Are we dealing with excessive or abnormal cellular growth (cancer) or decreased cellular function (possibly from changes associated with old age)? Is it an immune problem? If so, is it caused by something that is attacking the immune system from outside, or is your cat's body attacking his own immune system from the inside? Are outside toxins a possibility, or is Kitty's body simply unable to eliminate his daily production of internal waste products?

From the answers to these questions we would have information with which to select secondary herbs to help restore the whole body to normal. To continue the example above, if the urinary problem is infectious (caused by bacteria or viruses), we would want to prescribe herbs with antibiotic potential as well as herbs to enhance the immune system in general.

Step 3: Evaluate Other Factors

Are there any other factors that may be implicated in the whole disease — factors that we can help alleviate with herbs? For example, in nearly any disease, your cat will need to eliminate toxic products generated from tissue inflammation, loss of normal function, or infection. The body's primary organ for toxin elimination is the liver, so most of my herbal prescriptions include herbs that help liver function.

Step 4: Choose Facilitators

Are there any herbs that will facilitate the transport or delivery of other herbs to target organs? Cayenne, for example, acts to improve circulation in general, which helps move bioactive chemicals from herbs into areas where they are needed.

INCLUDING TONICS IN HEALTH CARE

According to Daniel P. Mowery, Ph.D., in *Herbal Tonic Therapies* (Keats Publishing, 1993), a tonic herb is any substance that balances the biochemical and physiological events that comprise body systems. *Homeostasis* is the word scientists use to describe this balance; *normality* and *equilibrium* are other frequently used terms for the same purpose. Keep in mind that a tonic does not just stimulate a body system; it acts to move the body back to an optimum state — stimulating or strengthening when necessary, or depressing, lowering, or relaxing when those actions are appropriate.

True tonic herbs also:
- Must be free of side effects
- Must have few or no contraindications
- Should be able to be consumed by cats in small amounts on a daily basis without adverse side effects (including addiction or tolerance)
- May exhibit bidirectional characteristics

A true tonic herb is recognized as such only after centuries of use by countless practitioners and patients.

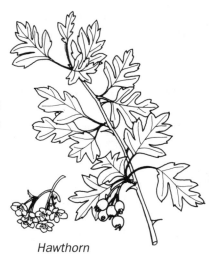
Hawthorn

SAFETY AND EFFICACY: SYNERGY AND BIDIRECTIONALITY

All medical practitioners judge the medicines they use by two specific criteria: safety and efficacy. Is the medicine reasonably safe to use on the majority of my patients? Can I expect positive results (good efficacy) most of the time? Herbs fulfill both of these criteria, and part of the reason they do is their ability to be both synergistic and bidirectional.

Understanding Synergy

As we've already noted, every herb contains a potpourri of bioactive chemicals. Many of these chemicals work together synergistically. This means that the total reaction of the plant's bioactive parts can be much more than the sum of its component parts.

When you give your cat a whole herb, he will benefit from the synergy of all its parts, and its overall efficacy will be enhanced. But if you give Buttons a pill that is a plant extract — that is, it contains only one of the plant's bioactive ingredients — then Buttons receives only the effects of that one active ingredient. This is not always bad, since we may want to produce a very specific action on the body. But in general, herbs are better used in toto; when the herb is used whole, all of the herb's bioactive ingredients work in synergy to positively affect your cat's entire body.

My Favorite Tonics

Here are some tonics I use in my veterinary practice:

- **Immune System:** Echinacea *(Echinacea* spp.), ginseng, astragalus *(Astragalus membranaceus),* licorice *(Glycyrrhiza glabra)*
- **Cardiovascular System:** Hawthorn *(Crataegus laevigata),* one of the "seaweeds," turmeric *(Curcuma longa),* motherwort *(Leonurus cardiaca),* Siberian ginseng *(Eleutherococcus senticosus),* valerian *(Valeriana officinalis)*
- **Nervous System:** Valerian, ginkgo *(Ginkgo biloba),* hop *(Humulus lupulus),* peppermint *(Mentha* x *piperita),* chamomile *(Anthemus nobilis; Matricaria recutita),* Siberian ginseng
- **Digestive System:** Milk thistle *(Silybum marianum),* artichoke *(Cynara scolymus),* dandelion *(Taraxacum officinale),* ginger *(Zingiber officinalis),* turmeric
- **Musculoskeletal System:** Alfalfa *(Medicago sativa),* devil's claw *(Harpagophytum procumbens),* yarrow *(Achillea millefolium),* saw palmetto *(Serenoa repens),* wild yam *(Dioscorea* spp.), echinacea, licorice, sarsaparilla *(Smilax* spp.*)*
- **Female Reproductive System:** Dong quai *(Angelica sinensis; A. polymorpha),* ginger, black haw *(Viburnum prunifolium),* cramp bark *(Viburnum opulis; V. trilobum),* valerian, raspberry *(Rubus idaeus),* licorice, black cohosh *(Cimicifuga racemosa),* chaste tree *(Vitex agnus-castus)*
- **Male Reproductive System:** Pygeum *(Pygeum africanum),* pumpkin seed *(Cucurbita pepo),* sarsaparilla, saw palmetto, Siberian ginseng

The Benefits of Bidirectionality

Bidirectionality means that a plant, via its many individual components, may direct its actions to one part or system of the body when needed but may have the opposite action if that is needed. Daniel Mowery refers to this as "specific hunger": the ability of animals and humans to select from a menu of foods containing nutrients the body is lacking at the time, thus restoring or maintaining homeostasis. Bidirectionality enhances herbal safety because the herbs help the body return to a balanced state. In addition, one herb can be used for many different diseases.

Ginseng, for instance, contains two bioactive ingredients: Rb ginsenosides and Rg ginsenosides. Each ingredient has an opposing action on blood pressure. Rb ginsenosides lower blood pressure, while Rg ginsenosides raise blood pressure. These opposing actions help balance blood pressure. Ginseng also contains components that raise and others that lower blood sugar. Hawthorn berries, like ginseng, tend to help normalize both high and low blood pressure.

To give another example, echinacea, with its ability to act in two opposing directions, brings almost every aspect of immune function under control. If your cat has a lower-than-normal white cell count, echinacea acts to increase production of white cells in the bone marrow. But if your cat's white cell count is high, echinacea decelerates the production of these cells.

Echinacea

Note that with any bidirectional herb, if we use a one-ingredient extract of the plant it will *not* have a bidirectional effect.

ECHINACEA AND IMMUNITY

In addition to its bidirectional effect on white cell production, echinacea also stabilizes the histamine-containing mast cell membrane in animals that have symptoms from allergies. This is contrary to most immune enhancers, which often sensitize the animal who has allergies.

HAVE HERBS BEEN SCIENTIFICALLY PROVEN TO WORK?

The answer to this question is an emphatic yes, but . . .

Science, good science, is nothing more — and nothing less — than the unbiased observation of phenomena. Sounds simple enough, but it isn't. If it were simple, we would be able to say that many medicinal herbs have been scientifically validated. After all, millions of users over eons should provide adequate testimony.

Furthermore, many of the medicinal uses of herbs have been validated through the most rigorous scientific testing. This testing uses studies in which randomly selected subjects are treated with either a placebo or an herb. The studies are "double-blind," meaning that neither the patient nor the doctor knows who receives the placebo and who receives the herb. Some herbs have been tested on animals, while others have been tested on humans. Still other tests have used both animal and human subjects.

But chances are that your veterinarian or physician has never seen those studies. Many have been conducted overseas and, for some reason, the community of healers in the United States tends to disregard anything that is not from within its own boundaries.

Whole Plants vs. Extracts

When used in whole rather than extracted form, herbs are incredibly safe medicines. Well-known tonic herbs produce almost no adverse reactions. Millions of users throughout the ages can't all be wrong.

But whenever we alter the original whole-plant package we can create trouble for our cats. Since extracts do not contain an herb's protective bidirectional ingredients, the one biochemical that has been extracted may be concentrated to a toxic level. Remember: Part of an herb's protective mechanism is that vast amounts of any one chemical are not usually concentrated in its leaves, roots, or flowers.

On the other hand, because most herbs lack huge concentrations of a specific bioactive substance, they often create a mild medicinal reaction in patients. Herbs usually act in subtle ways, and it may be weeks to months before you'll see any reaction in your cat. For my patients, especially for those with chronic conditions, I appreciate this slow and subtle reaction; "slow and easy" perfectly complements my other, specific medicines.

So keep in mind that if your cat has just been hit by a car or has endured some other type of trauma, you don't want to call an herbalist. *Do not hesitate* to take your cat to the veterinarian if an emergency situation arises.

What's more, many of the scientifically valid studies performed in the United States never reach the journals your veterinarian (or physician) reads; those journals are heavily funded by commercial pharmaceutical companies. As you can guess, these companies aren't wild about you being able to replace their expensive drugs with "weeds" from your backyard. So good scientific studies on herbs are not always easy to find.

And the problems run even deeper than that. Our reductionist model of medicine tries to boil down a disease to its smallest biochemical reason, and then it attempts to apply another chemical to "attack and cure" the problem. This mentality is only natural for scientists (and even some herbalists), who like to think that there is one bioactive chemical hidden within an herb or a drug that will cure a specific disease. But we've already seen that this does not apply to herbs, because they are plants with a veritable plethora of bioactive ingredients that act both synergistically and bidirectionally.

Cleavers

ARE DOUBLE-BLIND STUDIES REALLY THE ANSWER?

Even though double-blind studies really do not remove examiner bias, our scientists continue to insist on the double-blind study as their gold standard for testing. But not all herbs have been scientifically validated, and some of the most popular ones, such as kava kava, ginkgo, and ma huang, have not even withstood the scrutiny of time and trial. Because scientists insist on double-blind studies, they tend to ignore the practical, at-home trials that have been conducted for centuries by millions of people around the world. But even the most controlled scientific study cannot remove all of the outside factors that affect results, so we need to think in terms of whether a treatment is making the patient feel better. The simplest way to determine effectiveness is to ask yourself how bad your cat was doing before treatment. Then ask how he is doing after treatment. If there is improvement, the treatment is working effectively. If none; perhaps not. If he's getting worse, certainly not. In this way, you and your holistic vet can decide on the best course of treatment.

What is the concerned cat companion to do? Read on for some useful suggestions.

Find a Reputable Practitioner

The first step in successful herbal treatment is to find an herbalist or a holistic practitioner you can trust (see Resources for more information). Your trustworthy practitioner should have a good scientific background along with the horse sense to apply and then evaluate herbal medicines in clinical situations. Let the practitioner be the one to evaluate the scientific validity of claims made about an herb as well as clinical applications of that herb.

Choose Your Herbs Wisely

Use herbs that have been proven to be safe and effective over generations of use by multitudes of folks. Part 3 will give you a good base of herbs from which to choose. Whenever possible use the tonic herbs. Avoid what I call the designer herbs — those plants that are the current media darlings — until they have been around long enough to be properly evaluated in a clinical and scientific environment.

Become a Smart Consumer

Do not rely on media reports or on the stockperson in the health food or pet store for accurate information. Instead, refer to the Resources for good herbal magazines. Become knowledgeable about herbs and their specific uses; this book is an excellent start. After you complete your research, use the herbs for your cat's — and your — health. Practical application is the very best way to educate and empower yourself.

And if you feel you must have scientific validation for a particular herb, remember to

> *Y*ou'd be surprised how many of my clients bring me an herb sold to them by a store clerk, who has told them it would be good for their cat's problem. You'd probably not be surprised if I tell you that, nine times out of ten, the herb does not apply.

evaluate the studies that have used the *whole* herb, not an extracted biochemical.

Learning about Herbs

A t first glance, learning about herbs may seem an almost impossible task. There are, after all, thousands of herbs, and the medicinal aspects of herbology come packaged with foreign-sounding terminology and treatments. What's more, it often seems that each and every herb has dozens of practical, medicinal uses.

TIPS FOR YOUR HERBAL EDUCATION

Well, buck up, matey. You can make learning about herbs much easier on yourself by following a few practical tips. In fact, becoming acquainted with herbs can be the most enjoyable task you've ever undertaken. This chapter will tell you how to go about it.

Keep It Simple

Sure, there are several thousand medicinal herbs. So what? Do you need to know everything about all of them? Absolutely not! In fact, many of the traditional herbalists used only 10 to 12 herbs *total* in their entire practice. In a typical year I might use 30 to 40 herbs on a routine basis, with a very few more that I've added to help a rare patient — often after I've looked up and studied the seldom-used herb, just for that patient's special needs.

The Many Uses of Mullein

I began my herbal studies with mullein, *Verbascum thaspus*. Over the years, whenever I've come across any new information on mullein, I've added it to my personal "Book of Mullein Lore," which now contains several dozen pages. Mullein has taken me down roads of learning I've never been on before, and many are avenues I'd probably never have traveled had it not been for this fascinating herb.

For example, did you know that the "moly" Mercury gave Ulysses to use as a charm against Circe's enchantments was mullein? Well, I didn't, but this bit of lore encouraged me to read *The Odyssey* for the first time — which in turn began my fascination with the classics.

If you like historical trivia, you'll be interested to know that mullein was called the Herb of Love or Herbe of Protection in medieval times. In the seventh century the herb was so important it was named Herbe de St. Fiacre, after the Irish saint who became the patron saint of gardeners.

Mullein has long been thought to have both evil and good properties. One of its common names, hag's taper, refers to its supposed use as a transportation aid for witches in the days before broomsticks. Christian lore places mullein, or Heaven's Blaze, under Mary's protection, as per the saying "Our dear Lady travels the land, carrying Heaven's Blaze in her hand."

We can also learn more about an herb from its historical uses. Roman ladies used mullein flowers to dye their hair blond, and Mormon women rubbed the rough leaves on their cheeks to create a red flush. Native American people have used mullein seeds to paralyze fish (much like today's chemical rotenone), making the fish easy to gather as they float on the pond's surface.

Mullein is often thought of as a "protector plant." In olden days people hung mullein leaves in their home to keep negativity away, and they stuffed the herb into pillows to guard against nightmares. Even today European farmers refer to mullein as weathercandles, and they grow it close to their houses and outbuildings to keep lightning away.

Follow Your Interests

Herbs are truly the most fascinating study I've ever undertaken. Their medicinal aspect in animals is most interesting. But so, too, are some of the folktales that involve herbs, their appearance in literature and visual art, their historical uses in various cultures, and their mythical and magical properties. Whatever your special interests and fascinations, use them to ease your herbal learning curve. Remember that whenever we can attach a personal reason to our studies, the topic becomes much easier to learn.

Get to Know the Organ Systems

Perhaps you have a more intimate need to know about herbs. Maybe your cat has a heart condition, for example. There are many herbs that are heart helpful, and you could spend the next several months studying those herbs and how they affect the heart. From this study you could decide which ones would be best for Kitty's condition.

Join the Herb-of-the-Month Club

Nothing will drive learning better than a vital, personal need to know. But if your family is free of diseases at the present time, be happy and subscribe to the Herb-of-the-Month Club. Pick an herb — any herb — and take a month to study it. (Okay, you might be smarter than the rest of us, and you might be able to study two or three herbs every month, but be sure you do not bite off more herbs than you can chew. The secret is to really learn about one herb at a time.)

Learn the herb's Latin name (see the box on page 29), where it grows and what it looks like, which parts are used medicinally, its general actions on body systems, and any contraindications for usage. Then learn tidbits about the herb that will connect it to your special interests — stuff like its folklore, magical uses, special medicinal uses for female or male systems, and so forth.

By studying just one herb a month, in a few short years you'll know an awful lot about several dozen herbs.

ABOUT LATIN NAMES

Yeah, I know: They're a big pain in the brain. But, if you're going to be serious about herbal medicine (and herbs in general), you'll just have to grit your teeth and learn them. All medicinal uses are referenced to the Latin names of the plants, so there won't be any (potentially) fatal mistakes. There are simply too many species and too many common names, and this can be confusing unless you are familiar with the Latin names.

For example, I know of at least a dozen plants that are called snakeroot in one place or another. Here in Kansas, echinacea (*Echinacea* spp.), an immune-system balancer, is one of several plants known by that name. But I once had a traveling herbalist from Arizona try to sell me his local snakeroot, which was osha (*Ligusticum porteri*) — an herb used primarily for respiratory and intestinal problems. Had I purchased and used his snakeroot, my patients would have responded in an entirely different manner.

Insist on a Three-Book Minimum

If you are going to be serious about medicinal herbs, you'll need to own at least three good plant books. I own more than 500 herb books, and it seems I am constantly discovering some lovely little factoid about plants hidden within one of those books. And these little tidbits have ultimately helped me get to know — really know — the herbs.

Gone are the days when you couldn't find a decent herb book. Many of the herb books on the market today are good, if not excellent. (Of course, this one is the best of the best, but that goes without saying!) However, no one book can be complete in all it says about herbs, and no book can contain a complete listing of all medicinal plants. You will find invaluable information in almost any herbal book, and some of that material you won't be able to find in any other book.

In addition, books often contradict one other. When one book doesn't agree with another, I know that I need to do more research to find out which of the two has the better information. For example, one book might say that an herb is perfectly safe, while another lists three paragraphs of contraindications. In that case, I continue my research to weed out the incorrect information. I always wait until I have a thorough understanding of the herb before I use it on my patients.

Use It!

Now, there's book learning, and there's real learning. Real learning is hands on. Herbs are meant to be used. They were sent to earth so we mortals could learn to heal our pets and ourselves by using the healers we find in our own backyards.

Take it one herb at a time. Read about the herb, and then apply your knowledge. See how your cat likes it. Mix up a tea and soak his food in it. Try sprinkling the chopped herb over his food. Give him a bit of tincture and see how he takes to it. And while your cat tries the herb, take it yourself and see how it affects you.

Get Your Hands Dirty

Most of the healing herbs mentioned in this book can be grown in your own backyard. There's no better way to be intimately connected to the healing powers of Mother Earth than when your hands are in the soil/soul of healing, and you're getting dirty and sweaty while stretching, hoeing, pulling, and digging. Watch the herbs grow in the sun, and pick them for your family's use. You'll be learning all the while.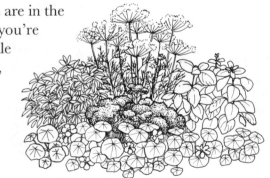

Let Nature Be Your Guide

Some of our most powerful healing herbs are known by many as weeds. But weeds have much to teach us.

Tis Mal Crow, a Native American healer friend of mine, claims that he can tell which disease will enter a family and when by observing the plants growing around the family's household. *Yeah, right,* I thought when I first heard the story.

But when I returned home to midtown Kansas City, I noticed a beautiful mullein plant growing in a neighbor's rock garden. It was the only mullein in the neighborhood, and I had tried, unsuccessfully, to grow the plant for years. So one afternoon I chatted with my neighbor about his new wife and mentioned how much I admired his wonderful mullein. He hadn't noticed the mullein, thought it was just another weed. But he told me that his wife was in the hospital being treated for asthma — one of the primary diseases mullein is used to treat. Aha.

Watch the weeds in your backyard. Perhaps they are trying to teach you something.

LEARNING *FROM* THE HERBS

Mullein is a favorite herb of mine because, thanks to a herd of deer, it was the first plant to really teach me about medicinal herbs. One blustery autumnal Kansas day I watched as a small herd of deer feasted on a rangy weed in our backyard. After they finished, I took out a weed identification book and, after much searching, I identified the herb as mullein. I thought it strange for the deer to concentrate on one weed when there were still many other green plants around. Once I'd tasted mullein's fuzzy, stick-to-the-roof-of-your-mouth leaves, I wondered even more.

After a little more research into the medicinal properties of mullein, I understood that the deer were simply preparing their lungs for the cold, wet weather to follow, and mullein was their protective herb of choice.

Make Your Herbal Studies Fun

Herbs — and herbalists — are a hoot. The more fun your studies, the more you'll learn.

Much like the soil they grow in, herbs are something you can really dig into. There's simply nothing more fascinating than herbs, and you can let your studies take you in whatever direction piques your interest. While this book focuses on medicinal applications of herbs in cats, there are virtually endless options to whet your special-interest appetite. Enjoy the adventure.

Delivery Systems

Some cats will naturally take to the herbs they need. For those individuals, using a tea or bulk herb on the food or in the water is the best dosing method. Others are not herb lovers, and they may take some additional coaxing. Capsules or tablets work well for stubborn critters, *if* you can get the pills down. (Many of them are horse-pill size!) Tinctures (especially the glycerin-based, nonalcoholic ones) are accepted by most pets, and a small dose — generally several drops, two or three times a day — is all that is needed.

The key is to use *whichever* herbal delivery method (bulk herbs, teas, tablets, capsules, or tinctures) works most easily for you and for your cat! Following is some more information to help in your selection.

DOSAGE AND POTENCY

How much of the herb do I give and for how long? Well, if I were to look at the herbs as a "Western medicine man," I would want to know what quantity of a specific chemical is needed to counter-attack the disease-causing biochemical entity that has invaded Kitty's body. Using Western medicine's paradigms I would be evaluating a drug's *potency* according to its biochemical constituents and how those constituents affect individual cells.

Then my therapeutic approach would be to build up a blood level of the single-entity drug to a point where it would be effective in most (but certainly not all) patients, and I would continue using that drug for a set amount of time, depending on the drug. Many practitioners simply ignore the potential for adverse side effects of the drug, putting them into the "reasonable costs for the benefits rendered" category.

As a holistic practitioner who uses herbs, however, I view the disease and the cure entirely differently. First of all, I must remember I am not using a single-entity drug that requires a specific blood level to be effective. Herbs have both synergy and bidirectionality working for them. Thus, from the perspective of therapeutic activity, trying to determine an herb's potency is nearly impossible, and it doesn't make much sense to try to do so by biochemical analysis. As an herbalist, I recognize that the most effective use of the herbs is to activate and rejuvenate an organ system (or multiple organ systems), so I will be looking for herbs — and supplements, medications, and other factors — to help bring the animal's whole body back into balance.

How much herb it will take to activate an organ system depends on the herb and the animal. Each individual disease and each individual animal will need a different amount of herb to return to normal health, or homeostasis.

Licorice

Dose to Effect

In light of all this, the easiest way to look at herbal dosages is to "give them to effect." My basic rule is to **start out slowly,** with low doses at first. Then, after a month or so, when the cat adjusts to her herbal intake, **taper off** or **add on,** depending on her reaction.

Now, there are exceptions to this general rule, but in my practice they are few and far between. When treating a bacterial infection, for example, I might want to ensure that the blood level of active antibacterial ingredients is high enough to be effective. In that case I would be concerned about the "standardized" level of the antibacterials in the herb. But even with a bacterial infection, for the long term I am much more concerned about enhancing the immune system than I am in confronting the bacteria by outside means. (It is interesting that plenty of evidence indicates that antibiotics commonly used in Western medicine, while they are combatting bacteria, actually have an adverse effect on the patient's overall immune system.)

Building on these ideas, here are some other suggestions and strategies for combining herbs in different ways, depending on what is most acceptable to your cat:

- **Expect slow, easy results.** Herbs most often need to be given for at least 30 days before you'll see appreciable results. Look for mild and subtle — *and* long-lasting — changes.
- **Use the delivery system that works best (and most easily) for your cat.** It is more important to get the herbs into her system than to worry about the "proper" way to dose.
- **Start out slow and then, depending on the cat's reaction, taper off or add on.** Often very small amounts of herb are enough to activate organ systems, ultimately leading to the cure you want.

GENERAL RULES FOR ADMINISTERING HERBS TO CATS

Follow these guidelines to determine how much of an herbal preparation you should give your cat.

Cat Weight	Sprinkles (put on Pet's food once daily)	Teas (pour over food or into Pet's water)	Capsules/ Tablets	Tinctures (in Pet's water or food or given directly by mouth)
1 to 5 lbs.	a very small pinch	⅛ cup once daily	small chip tablet or ⅛ to ¼ capsule* 1 to 2 times daily	1 to 3 drops 1 to 3 times daily
5 to 10 lbs.	a small pinch	⅛ to ¼ cup 1 to 2 times daily	¼ to ½ capsule** 1 to 2 times daily	3 to 5 drops 1 to 3 times daily
10 to 20 lbs.	a bigger pinch	¼ cup 1 to 2 times daily	½ to 1 capsule** 1 to 3 times daily	3 to 5 drops 1 to 3 times daily
Over 20 lbs.	2 pinches to 1 teaspoon	¼ to ⅓ cup 1 to 2 times daily	½ to 1 capsule** 2 to 4 times daily	5 to 10 drops 1 to 3 times daily

* Open capsule and remove powder.

** Or tablet.

SELECTING HERBS

In my experience, the best benefits are obtained with top-quality whole herbs. Most important to me is that the herbs are organically grown; pesticides and herbicides can interfere with the healing properties of plants. I don't find a huge difference between fresh and dried herbs, especially when top-quality products are used.

A good herbal wholesale outlet store uses numerous levels of quality control to ensure that the plants they sell are of the highest potency. A quality-control manager will conduct a physical examination of the herbs — look at them, smell them, feel them. He may also perform a chemical analysis, determine the spore content under a microscope, and even send a sample out for spectral chromatography. But it's just as important that the manager perform a simple taste test to ensure positive identification of the herb!

The best advice I can give for buying herbs is to find a source you trust and stick with it. There is a huge herb store not far from where I live, but I found out recently that the herbs are warehoused in a building that is regularly fumigated! On the other hand, I found an herbal outlet in Iowa (Frontier Herbs; see Resources) that offers plant materials that are consistently very fresh and well prepared. I now use that outlet for almost all my herbs.

What to Look for in Dried Herbs

When selecting dried herbs I look for plants that are still resilient. If the plant is so brittle that it falls apart at a touch, it's probably too old to be useful. I also look for plants that retain a lot of color; properly dried green plants are still bright green. If the plants are brown and the leaves are crunchy, they are too old.

What to Look for in Fresh Herbs

When buying fresh herbs, select fresh-smelling plants that look healthy and have strong green leaves. Avoid plants that are dusty or browned or whose leaves have a moth-eaten appearance.

I often gather wild herbs for use on my animals and me. You can do this, too, but you *must* adhere to these cautions:

- **Accurate identification is critical,** for obvious reasons. Most of the herbs I recommend are very common and easy to identify. But until you are intimately familiar with an herb you should have an expert confirm your identification.

- **Be careful about harvesting herbs in urban and suburban environments,** which have most likely been treated with pesticides and herbicides. Even plants within a certain distance — some say 300 feet — from rural roads are not safe. Roadside plants, as well as herbs that grow near railroads and under high-voltage power lines, are typically sprayed with potent chemicals. Do not use an herb unless you are absolutely certain it has not been sprayed.

How to Store Herbs

If you've purchased fresh herbs, use them within a few days of purchase; they will spoil eventually, just like food. If you've purchased dried herbs, you can store them for later use. Put your dried herbs in separate clean glass jars and cap them tightly. Don't forget to label each jar with the name of the herb and the date you purchased it. Keep the containers out of direct light and heat, and the herbs will last for several months.

BULK HERBS

There are three ways to use bulk herbs:

1. Make a tea by simmering or steeping the fresh or freshly dried herbs in water.
2. Use tea bags as a more convenient way to make teas.
3. Sprinkle the bulk herb over your pet's food, much as you would add salt to your own meal.

When adding an herbal taste to Tiger's food or water, be sure he continues to eat and drink. In general, teas seem to be more readily accepted than sprinkles, at least at first.

Using Sprinkles

Many, but not all, cats enjoy the taste of herbs. (My favorite example is cayenne, or red pepper, which I've discovered is a preferred seasoning for many of my patients, feline and canine.) Grind the herbs into bite-sized pieces before using — coffee grinders work well. Try the sprinkles on a small portion of your cat's food, and see whether he selects or avoids that portion of his serving. Evidence suggests that it is important for the animal to taste the herb; tasting evidently triggers other body systems to actively accept the herb's healing properties.

Pros and Cons of Bulk Herbs

There are big advantages to bulk herbs *if* your pet is accustomed to their taste:

- They are low in cost.
- They are easy to administer.
- They activate the taste buds (see above).
- The whole herb is present, adding bidirectionality and synergistic effects (see page 20).
- There is no concentration of one ingredient with possible harmful, single-ingredient doses present.

There are also certain disadvantages:

- Not all health food stores carry bulk herbs.
- Those that do may not pay attention to shelf life.
- Some bulk herbs may have been sprayed (at the farm, warehouse, or distribution center) with potentially toxic pesticides.
- Not all pets enjoy the taste of herbs. However, it's been my experience that most adapt to the taste, given a few months' time.

Using Teas

After brewing tea with fresh or dried herbs (see recipe on page 38) and then cooling the liquid, pour a small quantity onto your cat's food or into his water several times a day.

Don't let the herbalist jargon of tisane, decoction, and infusion befuddle you. If you're making a tea from thick, fibrous stuff, such as a root stalk, boil it a little harder and longer to make a **decoction.** If you're making your tea from fragile, sweet-smelling herbal flowers or leaves, hold that fragrance in by covering your pot and boiling lightly. Voilà, you've made a **tisane** or **infusion.**

If you're a simple person from Kansas, like I am, you just boil some water, pour it over the plant stuff, and let it sit in a covered teapot until it's steeped for however much time you have available.

Basic Herbal Tea

8 tablespoons fresh herb *or* 4 teaspoons freshly
   dried bulk herb *or* 2 herbal tea bags
1 quart water

1. Simmer or steep the fresh or freshly dried bulk herb or tea bags
   for 10 to 20 minutes. Strain out the herb material and allow the
   liquid to cool.
2. Pour ⅛ to ¼ cup or so of tea over your cat's food 2 or 3 times a
   day, or add small amounts to his water.
3. Store excess tea in the refrigerator to use over the next few days.

TINCTURES (A.K.A. LIQUID OR FLUID EXTRACTS)

These preparations are made by soaking the fresh or freshly dried
herb in a solvent. In general, tinctures are considered more clinically effective than capsules
or tablets.

There are two major sol-
vents: alcohol and glycerin
(or glycerite). For most herbs
alcohol is the best solvent,
since it extracts more of the
plant's ingredients than
other solvents. Alcohol, however, can be toxic in some
patients, causing gastro-
intestinal irritation, allergic
reactions, and (at least in
people) habituation.

> *If you have used fresh plants,
> you may find a gooey kind of
> scum — a viscous layer where
> the water and the oil haven't
> mixed — on the top of your
> extract. Don't worry a bit about
> it; there is nothing harmful about
> this layer. In fact, I know one
> herbalist who swears this gooey
> stuff is the most potent part
> of the tincture!*

Nonalcoholic (often found on the shelves as "pediatric") tinctures
are typically extracted in glycerin, a sweet-tasting solvent that can
mask the taste of bitter herbs. Glycerin, which is available in most
health food stores, is not quite as efficient as alcohol at extracting
plant constituents, but it is a good alternative. *Note:* Cats can have
trouble assimilating alcohol (it is said that they lack the enzyme necessary to metabolize it), so glycerin is always the preferred solvent for
making tinctures for cats.

All you need to make a tincture is a clean jar with a tight-fitting lid, as much herb as it will take to fill the jar (fresh and dried herbs may be used with equal success), and glycerin to cover the herbs.

Tinctures are simple to make and last for long periods.

Administering Tinctures

Tinctures can be used on your cat's food or in small amounts in his water. Or for the fastidious eater, you can use an eyedropper to squirt a few drops into his mouth or into the fold at the crease of his lips. Whenever possible use the non-alcoholic tinctures. I have found that often very small amounts — a few drops between the lower lip and gums at the side of the cat's mouth 2 or 3 times daily, plus a few more drops in his water or atop his food — are more than enough to be effective. Pet and praise and feed your cat a little treat afterward so that she will associate positive experiences with the administration of the tincture.

Simple Tincture

Fresh or dried herb of choice
Vegetable glycerin
1. Stuff a clean glass jar with the herb; leave 1 to 2 inches of space at the top. Then fill the jar with glycerin.
2. Close the jar tightly and put it in a dark cupboard for 1 to 2 weeks. Shake it every few days.
3. Strain the plant material out of the liquid. Muslin or cheesecloth works best to capture all the little plant particles, and you can also use the cloth to squeeze as much liquid as possible from the plants. Rebottle the liquid and discard the plant material. Label the bottle with the date and the plant and solvent used. Glycerin tinctures will keep longer in the refrigerator. Do not expose the tincture to direct heat or light.

GIVING A CAT A TINCTURE

Hold your cat securely. At the side of his mouth, gently pull down his lower lip.

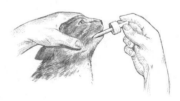

Use the eyedropper to squeeze a few drops of tincture between the lower lip and gum. The easiest place is usually the corner of the mouth, right where the upper and lower lips meet.

CAPSULES AND TABLETS

There are two basic ways to make capsules and tablets:

1. Pack the powdered form of the herb (along with various fillers) into a capsule.
2. Use a tincture of the herb, evaporate water and alcohol, and place the substance on a powdered binder to form the tablet.

Capsules and tablets are inexpensive, and for the easy-to-pill cat they are convenient to give. On the downside: Adulteration may be a problem since the powdered forms are difficult to identify. Some herbal capsules contain as much as 65 percent filler, such as soy powder or millet powder. And some commonly used binding agents include magnesium stearate, which can come from either animal or vegetable sources, and dicalcium phosphate, which may contain lead. It pays to know your herbal manufacturer and distributor.

Using Capsules and Tablets

If it is a product made for animals, read the label; if it is a made-for-humans product, read the label and adapt the dosage to your cat's size (see the box on page 44). Capsules and tablets are not my favorite way to administer herbs, but if they are the only way to get Kitty to take his medicine, then have at it. Rule #1 applies here: Whatever works.

GIVING A CAT A PILL

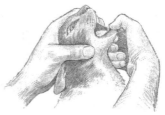

Restrain the cat and grip the upper jaw over the top of his head. Apply light pressure to his upper gums and gently pull up. You can also use the scruffing technique (see the box on page 41), then tilt the cat's head up and slightly back.

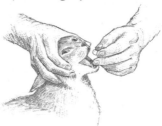

Place the pill on the very back of the tongue (past the "hump") with your other hand. Do this as quickly as possible.

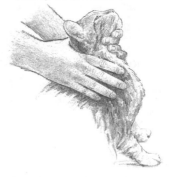

Hold the cat's mouth shut with one hand while stroking his throat to encourage him to swallow.

TOPICAL HERBAL APPLICATIONS

There must be hundreds of topical herbal medicines on the market — oils, ointments, salves, soaps, and so forth. Skin is an animal's largest body organ, and it readily and actively absorbs all sorts of healing agents. Topical use of herbs, then, can be a highly effective delivery system for herbal healing.

We need to be a mite careful when using the topicals, however, because some of the carrying agents may be irritating to Pet's skin. Also, cats will almost certainly lick off anything applied to their skin, and some of the carrying agents may cause intestinal upset.

ABOUT RESTRAINING CATS

Cat restraint can be a piece of cake . . . or a real challenge. Some cats will respond to very light restraint, and they will let you do whatever you need to do as long as you have a calm and gentle touch. For these cats the curl-into-a-ball technique may be best. Place your cat on your lap or in the corner of his favorite couch. Make him comfortable with gentle words and caresses and gradually get him into as tight a ball as possible, with all four feet snugly underneath his body. Cats in this position will often accept medicines or other treatments as long as you are gentle and reassuring.

Most cats can be restrained with what we call "scruffing." With a firm hold on the loose skin over the lower neck and shoulders, firmly but gently lift up, raising Cat's front feet so they are free in the air. This may sound a bit drastic, but remember that this is what Momma Cat does to her young whenever she moves them. Most cats will calm down so long as you maintain the hold.

Other cats will tolerate no restraint, and my advice with these is to *not* fight them. Try another way to administer the herbs — small amounts hidden in a favorite food, for example, or as a tea drizzled over their food. If Cat really hates one herb, ask your herbalist or holistic vet for an alternative. The beauty of herbal medicines is that alternatives are always available.

How to Choose Topicals

Natural-based oils and salves — such as beeswax; lanolin; and coconut, olive, almond, grapeseed, and jojoba oils — are best and cause the fewest reactions. Petroleum-based and coal tar–based products seem to cause more reactions, and if the product label contains something you can't pronounce, don't use it. If your cat is especially sensitive to almost anything, use a test dose — a small amount applied to one area of your cat's skin — and watch for adverse reactions for 4 to 6 hours.

Making Your Own Topicals

My favorite topical application for wounds or other small areas is an herbal spritz. First make the appropriate herb into a tea (see page 38 for instructions), then allow it to cool, and spritz it onto the area directly. Use this treatment 3 to 5 times a day. The spritzed herb will dry quickly, giving your cat little reason to lick. And even if he does lick, he ingests only the healing herb.

Remember too that because herbs are absorbed so readily through the skin, a daily romp and roll in your herbal garden is one of the best ways to apply the healing qualities of the herbs.

A special cautionary note: In some instances I find the use of herbal aromatherapy to be very effective. But individual herbal constituents of the essential oils used in aromatherapy may be concentrated to levels dozens of times higher than those found in the original herbs. With the altered levels of individual herb constituents we may increase the possibility of adverse reactions, especially if your cat can lick and ingest the essential oil. So I limit topical application of essential oils to those herbs I know are nontoxic, and I apply only small amounts (a drop or two will do) to the rear of the cat's neck, just behind the ears.

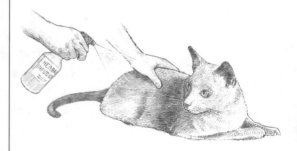

USING AN HERBAL SPRITZ

Spray the cooled infusion directly on the affected area.

STANDARDIZED EXTRACTS

Standardized extracts have been certified by the manufacturer — usually using stringent laboratory methods, such as liquid chromatography — to contain the stated amount of specific constituents. Standardizing may provide more consistency in potency and help ensure that the correct plant is being sold.

There are two types of standardized extracts:

• **Whole-plant standardized extracts,** in which the entire plant is extracted and the plant's constituents are guaranteed to be present in amounts above a certain level. For instance, a capsule might be guaranteed to contain exactly one milligram of the herb. But if only the amount of the herb present in the product is guaranteed, you have no idea of the potency.

• **Purified standardized extracts,** which are herbal extracts made with a variety of solvents, with the active ingredient(s) removed from the parent plant. In this way, the original balance of the herb is significantly altered, as one constituent is "pumped up" above its normal levels. A St.-John's-wort capsule, for example, might contain 0.5 milligram of hypericin, which is commonly believed to be the herb's active ingredient. But this method assumes that the hypericin is the biochemical constituent that is needed, and the body doesn't get the benefits of the plant's other active ingredients.

There are plenty of out-to-make-a-buck-at-any-cost herbal hooligans, perfectly willing to extract your dollars for an inferior product. It is not uncommon to find herbal products on the market that do not contain (or that contain only minuscule amounts of) the herbs advertised on the package label. So some form of quality assurance is needed.

Are Standardized Extracts the Best Choice?

I am not so certain that standardization is the answer. Any standardization process neglects the all-important healing factors involved in the synergistic actions of the *numerous* active ingredients of all herbal medicines. In addition, standardization typically looks at only the chemical properties of one part of the herb, again neglecting the possibility that the whole herb may have more potential value than is contained in its chemical constituents.

Finally, standardization does not take into account factors that may be important in the herb's potency and, thus, the overall healing properties, such as method of harvest, time of harvest, sex of the plant (or other individual conditions of the plant), organic or commercial growing conditions, and so forth.

To my way of thinking, standardization is a lazy way of letting others (the government) do what should really be the herbalist's groundwork of finding trustworthy herbal farmers, producers, suppliers, and distributors. Remember that when you grow (or wild-craft) and make your own herbal medicines, *you* become the most trustworthy one. And you'll know that by using the whole herb, rather than altering the ratio of the biochemicals naturally present, you won't risk losing the synergy and bidirectionality of the plant.

ADAPTING HUMAN PRODUCTS FOR USE ON CATS

If what you've purchased is a product meant for humans, read the label and adapt the directions to your cat's size. Assume that an average human weighs 150 pounds. Here are some examples of how this works.

Tinctures. The label instructions on the human product are to give 15 to 30 drops, 3 to 4 times a day, for a total daily human dose of 45 to 120 drops. Your cat weighs 10 pounds. 10 = 1/15 of 150 pounds. She should receive 3 to 8 drops daily, preferably divided into 3 or 4 doses. A three-times-daily dosage, then, would be 1 to 3 drops per dose.

Capsules or tablets. The label instructions for humans are to give 3 to 5 capsules, 3 times a day. If your cat weighs 30 pounds (30 lbs. = 1/5 of the "normal" 150-pound human), you could give up to one capsule or tablet 3 times a day. But if your cat weighs only 15 pounds, you could break the tablet in two (or open the capsule and use about half of its contents) and use this dose 3 times daily.

Teas. Simmer fresh or dried bulk herb or an herb tea bag (see recipe on page 38). The tea will last for a few days in the refrigerator. Give your cat about 1/4 cup on her food 2 or 3 times a day.

part 2

Herbs for Organs, Systems, and Special Conditions

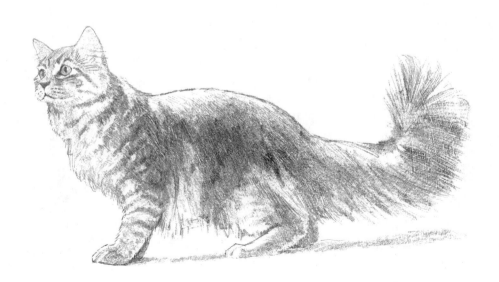

The Aging Body

I think cats age more gracefully than other animals. I mean, here I am, a 50-something graybeard, with rusty joints that make it a bit of a struggle just to get out of bed in the morning. I can't seem to maintain my weight, I don't hear as well as I once did, and I'm a lot slower in my get-along. My dog, Rufus, has paralleled me in all of these age-related changes, but my cats, Quixote and Little Cat, who are both the same age as Rufus, don't look or act any older than they did many years ago.

But the fact is that nearly all of the cats' body systems are not what they once were. And while the cats may not show their age as much as Rufus and I do, there's no denying that they are going through changes, too. They are not kittens anymore, and even if they don't know it or show it, their organs are not functioning quite as well, their eyesight is beginning to dim, their joints are starting to lose their flexibility, and their minds aren't as sharp as they once were. Nevertheless, all of us — Little Cat, Quixote, Rufus, and I — are learning that herbal tonics are the perfect companions as we continue our journey along the aging trail.

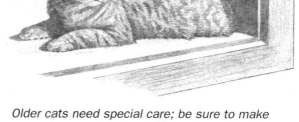

Older cats need special care; be sure to make note of any changes in their condition or behavior.

A HOLISTIC PROTOCOL FOR AGING

Nothing can prevent aging, but you can prevent some of the problems associated with this natural process. My cats and I take our daily dose of herbs for one organ system or the other. We'll use several of my favorite herbs (many of which are listed in this book), concentrating on one organ system for a month or so and then moving on to another. Over the years, all of us have come to enjoy the tart taste of the herbs; indeed, none of us enjoys our food quite as much without the tang of herbs sprinkled on top.

Evaluating Aging Organ Systems

I recommend a special annual exam for healthy geriatric cats, starting soon after they have passed their seventh or eighth birthday. Along with a regular physical exam, I suggest a complete blood count (CBC), a urinalysis, a series of blood chemistries, and possibly X rays. These exams are a way for me to screen for organ-related problems; catching these problems early, at a time when we can actually do something about them, is very important. The annual exam is the perfect way to identify organ systems that could be helped with herbs.

Use Tonic Herbs

Tonic herbs support the function of different organs; this, in turn, improves the overall health of the body. I prefer to use tonic herbs on an on/off basis, alternating them as dictated by our taste buds, our perceived needs for the month, and the availability of the herbs. My favorite tonic herbs for the aging cat include:

- **Echinacea,** a general immune-system balancer
- **Hawthorn,** a cardiotonic that helps the aging heart
- **Ginger,** which boosts a lethargic digestive system
- **Milk thistle,** a liver-function enhancer
- **Nettle,** a gentle, whole-body tonic
- **Dandelion,** which enhances liver function and is a diuretic
- **Bladderwrack,** a thyroid helper

Get Adequate Exercise

I am a firm believer in the adage "use it or lose it." Fortunately, your cats can be outside with you during the day, or you can play indoors with Kitty's favorite toys to give him the exercise he needs. Our cats seem to enjoy following us around as we do our chores on the farmstead. They probably get more exercise than the average cat; perhaps this is one of the reasons they are aging so gracefully.

Incorporate Antioxidants

As we age, our cells are producing more and more free radicals — chemicals that speed the aging process. One of the keys to anti-aging is to counter this overproduction of free radicals with antioxidants. Vitamins A and C are good antioxidants, but so too are many herbs. Some of the culinary herbs even have antioxidant activity. These include:

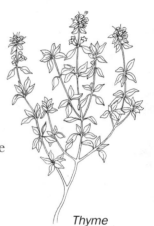

Thyme

- Oregano *(Origanum vulgare)*
- Basil *(Ocimum basilicum)*
- Thyme *(Thymus vulgaris)*

LONGEVITY HERBS

In addition to the above regimen, the cats, Rufus, and I are gradually adding to our daily intake herbs that can enhance the length and quality of life during the golden years.

Ginkgo (Ginkgo biloba)

Ginkgo is our primary anti-aging herb. It acts on two major systems of the body: the nervous system and the cardiovascular system. Ginkgo has proven effective in treating Alzheimer's disease, depression, and senile dementia. (In animals, senile dementia associated with Alzheimer's-like symptoms is referred to as cognitive dysfunction or dimming mind syndrome.) Ginkgo enhances both long-term and short-term memory in kittens and old critters alike.

This popular herb improves circulation and has good antioxidant activity. Studies also indicate that ginkgo is often effective for age-related hearing and vision loss, dizziness and vertigo, and tinnitus (ringing in the ear).

Rosemary (Rosmarinus officinalis)

A common culinary herb, rosemary contains bioactive ingredients that help prevent the breakdown of the chemical acetylcholine in the brain. A deficiency in acetylcholine is believed to be a contributing factor in senility in general and Alzheimer's disease in particular. Rosemary is also an important antioxidant.

> *Our pets, Little Cat, Quixote, and Rufus, and my wife and I all take our antiaging herbs on a daily basis, and I am firmly convinced that they are helpful. And judging by the comments from my many clients who are using the herbs I've recommended for their older dogs, herbs are truly one of the very best treatments available for the aging body.*

Turmeric (Curcuma longa)

Turmeric is the yellow component of curry powder, and it stimulates the liver's bile production. This herb is a potent antioxidant. Turmeric is also heart healthy, acting as a blood thinner (which prevents clots) and helping to prevent excess cholesterol accumulation.

Flaxseed Oil (Linum usitatissimum)

The oil from this plant is an excellent source of omega-3 fatty acids, the good fats that lower cholesterol, reduce triglycerides (which, along with cholesterol, are artery blockers), and prevent blood clots.

Green Tea (Camellia sinensis)

The green variety of tea contains flavonoids and polyphenols, which may be a more powerful antioxidant than vitamins C or E. Green tea is oxidized for a shorter period of time than black tea; the black variety does not have the same health benefits.

Gotu Kola (Centella asiatica)

A traditional herb of both Chinese and Ayurvedic medicine, gotu kola has antioxidant activity that protects the body from damage by free radicals. The herb is particularly useful for stress-related disorders and memory problems.

Arthritis and the Musculoskeletal System

Arthritis (and its cousin rheumatism) is a catchall term that encompasses several dozen disease states of the joints and other surrounding tissues, such as tendons, ligaments, cartilage, joint sacs (or bursae), muscles, and connective tissues. There are many conditions that cause arthritis and rheumatism, including infection (bacterial, viral, fungal, and parasitic), trauma, immune-mediated conditions, age-related changes, orthopedic surgery, and genetic factors. Each of these causes of arthritis has its own preferred method of treatment, so it is important to get an accurate diagnosis from your vet.

THE MUSCULOSKELETAL SYSTEM

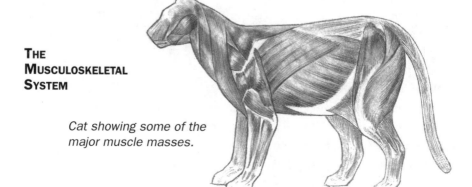

Cat showing some of the major muscle masses.

A BRIEF INTRODUCTION
TO ARTHRITIS AND HOLISTIC CARE

I have found that a holistic approach for treating the broad cate-gory of arthropathies is quite simply the best way to address this multifaceted disease. I get much better results now than I ever did with Western medicines, using a combined protocol of good nutri-tion, nutritional supplements, massage, passive exercise, and the alternative medicines of acupuncture, chiropractic, and herbs. Best of all, by using a holistic approach I see *far* fewer adverse side effects.

However, the caveats that apply to the use of alternative medi-cines for any disease apply even more in the case of arthritis:

- Each and every case presents a different picture of symp-toms, and the individual patient's symptoms will dictate what medicines should be used. In other words, there is no magic formula, herbal or otherwise, that will treat all arthritis cases.
- Alternative holistic methods do not typically work as fast as the whistle-and-bell remedies of Western medicine. Figure on at least two to three months and perhaps several different treatments before you'll see any appreciable results. In other words, there is no quick fix in alternative medicines. Remember that the trade-off here is that, in the long run, your cat will have far fewer negative side effects.
- Each pet has its own unique way of responding to treatments. Unfortunately, I have never been able to predict which patients will be the ones to respond. Again, alternative medi-cines do not offer a quick fix or magic formula.

Symptoms of Arthritis

When I first started using alternative medicines, I was surprised at the number of cats who were severely arthritic. Once I began to pay more attention to spine and joint mobility, I could easily discern an arthritic cat. Considering that most cats are paragons of the "couch potato" lifestyle, I guess I should not have been surprised.

In many cases, the owner of the arthritic cat is also surprised to hear that his cat has arthritis. After all, how would you know a cat has sore joints if all she does is lie around all day? On reflection, however, most owners are able to remember when their cat was able to move about more easily, and they can often relate the gradual decline in his ability to move with ease.

The most common feline arthritic problems I see in my practice are a potpourri of osteoarthritic arthropathies (characterized by degeneration of the articular cartilage, bone spurs at the edges of the joints, and changes in the synovial membrane that surrounds the joints) and degenerative arthropathies (characterized by deterioration of the joint cartilage, often accompanied by bone growth at the edges of the joints). The typical patient is five or more years old. The lower back (lumbar region) and hips are the most commonly affected areas. Occasionally I'll detect arthritis in other joints, but this is relatively rare and can usually be related to some past trauma.

In contrast to dogs, whose arthritic problems are, in my opinion, mostly induced by genetic structural abnormalities, I think cats develop arthritic changes as a result of their sedentary lifestyles. Joints need movement — flexion, extension, and rotation — to stay "well-oiled" and healthy. In contrast, joints that are not moved tend to lose their normal fluidity. A stagnated joint may begin to tighten, and eventually bone deposits may form.

Typically, the symptoms slowly get worse until the cat is having a difficult time getting up stairs or jumping onto Mom's bed. Your cat may cringe or even cry when you rub its back, and the back muscles may feel hotter than other muscles in the cat's body. You may notice that your cat seems to walk with a hunched back; pain causes muscle tension in the back, and this muscle tenseness often creates a noticeable lump of tightened muscles. There may be enough pain and inflammation over the cat's back or in his joints that you can see a noticeable limp when he walks, and sometimes individual joints are actually swollen. X rays may or may not demonstrate noticeable changes in joints and bony surfaces, but chiropractic evaluation often reveals joints that are less flexible than normal.

From the get-go I tell folks to figure on a minimum of 3 to 6 months of treatment before we'll see any appreciable results. But, once we do see results, they can be long lasting — and we will not be using any drugs that can actually be damaging.

Step 1: Acupuncture and Chiropractic

I feel that acupuncture and chiropractic are essential elements in any treatment regimen for arthritis. Typically, after several initial treatments the cat exhibits much less pain, and we almost always see partial or nearly complete return of function. I see such good results with acupuncture and chiropractic that I think it is just plain bad medicine — perhaps even malpractice — *not* to use them.

Step 2: Nutrition

Often a change in diet will be enough to relieve arthritic symptoms. Feed your cat wholesome, organic foods that are not over-processed and contain no synthetic preservatives, pesticides, herbicides, hormones, or artificial flavors or colorings.

Feverfew

Step 3: Supplements

There is a veritable stewpot of supplements that have worked seemingly miraculous results in some patients with arthritis. The two most important categories are chondroprotective agents and antioxidants.

Chondroprotective agents promote new cartilage growth and thus decrease pain and improve joint mobility. Glucosamine HCl products have generally given my patients the most consistent results. Other chondroprotective agents that I have tried include chondroitin sulfate, MSM (methylsulphonylmethane), and SAM-e (S-adenosylmethionine). I add these to my protocol when glucosamine hasn't seemed to work after a few months' trial. I use the regular human dosage schedule, altered to fit my feline patient's weight (see the box on page 44).

Antioxidants protect cells from damage caused by free radicals. Free radicals are produced when a cell is exposed to any of a number of toxins, including pesticides, herbicides, and toxic emissions in the air. Free radicals, which can damage and even destroy cells, are also produced by cells surrounding the joint whenever excess or abnormal strains or pressures are applied — for example, when the weight-bearing surfaces are out of normal alignment because of a skeletal disfigurement common in many of our nonfunctional, bred-to-look-funny-or-cute breeds. To put antioxidants to work on the disease, I add therapeutic (i.e., high) levels of vitamins A, C, and E — along with selenium — to the cat's diet for 3 to 6 months, and then decrease the dosage to protective levels. Check with your holistic vet for the proper dosage, which should be adjusted for the cat's size and the severity of the disease.

Herbal antioxidants. Many herbs are highly antioxidant and also contain good levels of necessary vitamins. I especially like the culinary herbs, including oregano *(Origanum vulgare)*, thyme *(Thymus vulgaris)*, ginger *(Zingiber officinalis)*, basil *(Ocimum basilicum)*, parsley *(Petroselinum crispum)*, and celery seed *(Apium graveolens)*, because they can be sprinkled on your cat's food daily — much as you would season your own dinner. Find a combination of these herbs along with cayenne and turmeric (see Step 5 for more information) that your cat will eat. It has been my experience that unless the cat has become completely spoiled with the pap that characterizes typical commercial pet foods, he'll enjoy one or more of these culinary treats.

OTHER ANTIOXIDANTS

In addition to the antioxidants listed, several others may prove helpful, including:

- SOD (superoxide dismutase)
- Glutathione peroxidase
- Dl methionine
- Pycnogenol

Other nutrients that have shown some promise in treating arthritis include:

- Niacinamide (vitamin B_3)
- Pyridoxine (vitamin B_6)
- Magnesium
- Manganese
- Copper
- Boron
- Zinc

In addition, the omega-3 fats found in deep-sea fish, flaxseed oil *(Linum usitatissimum),* and purslane *(Portulaca oleracea)* may also be helpful.

Step 4: Exercise and Massage

I am of the "use it or lose it" school of thinking, and the research on arthritis supports this approach. The more you can keep your cat moving and flexing his joints, the better. But there's your challenge: how do you get Kitty off the couch? Be creative.

Does your cat like catnip? If so, sprinkle it in places where he has to walk or jump to get to it. Play chase-the-artificial-mouse if that's one of your cat's favorite amusements. Put her food dish in a place where she has to walk to get to it. Take time for a supervised daily romp in the backyard. In short, do whatever you can to get your cat to be more active.

A daily light massage can also ease aches and pains as well as increase general body circulation. Now, there are some cats who want to be rubbed *only* on their time frame, when they darn well want to be rubbed. For these guys and gals, you'll probably need to limit your massage to times when it is okay with Cat. And a few cats just plain don't want to be rubbed or petted at any time, no way. Massage may not be the thing for these loners, although even the loners will usually pick a time and place when it's okay for you to rub and pet, as long as you are gentle.

Over the years I've seen several cats who really hate to be touched in a particular part of the body, or along a certain area of the back. Almost always — especially when the sore spots have not always been there — these areas are related to a "kink" in the spine, or an area of painful arthritis. This condition responds well to chiropractic adjustments, perhaps with added acupuncture and herbal medicines.

Massage is a great tool for reducing everyday aches and pains.

For many arthritic cats, however, even light exercise can be painful. If this is the case, see Step 5.

Step 5: Herbal Pain Relief

Pain and inflammation are common results of arthritic changes in the joint. But because it is most important to keep your cat on the go (see above), we need to do all we can to make her comfortable while moving. Herbs can be very helpful in relieving arthritis-related symptoms.

Licorice *(Glycyrrhiza glabra)* is an herb I commonly use to replace the anti-inflammatory action of the steroids that I once used in my Western medicine practice. (We have a saying in Western veterinary medicine: "No animal should die without having been treated with cortisone." So Western vets — including me in my past life — use steroids for *everything*.) It's nice to have a nontoxic option to steroids, so a good many of my patients receive a licorice root prescription. It may take a month or two before your cat displays positive results, but he'll avoid the adverse side effects of cortisone.

I am not convinced we ever see in our animals the high blood pressure problems we see in people who take prolonged, large doses of licorice root. But, to be honest, we never measure blood pressure in cats, so I can't be sure. I can say that I have used the herb on hundreds of dogs and cats, many with preexisting heart problems, and I haven't seen any cardiac or renal problems.

Cayenne *(Capsicum* spp.), taken internally, seems to offer pain relief for some patients. In addition, cayenne acts as a systemic stimulant, helping move herbs and other medicines into joint areas where they are needed. I am surprised by how many of my animal patients (both cats and dogs) enjoy the taste of cayenne sprinkled over their food, making this herb a great treatment option. In people, cayenne is also used topically as an ointment; it is applied directly over painful joints. However, our feline critters often go crazy trying to lick everything off their hair and skin, so they aren't usually good candidates for topical ointments that cause a bit of stinging.

Willow bark *(Salix* spp.) is rich in anti-inflammatory salicylates. Remember that the drug aspirin also contains salicylates, which have proven to be harmful in cats. Willow bark is not a single-entity drug, however, and it has the advantage of containing only small amounts of salicylates. It also has the advantage of bidirectionality (see page 20). While I am cautious in recommending willow bark for cats, I have not had problems using it, and it has apparent pain-relieving effects in some cats.

Other valuable herbs are:

- Wild yam *(Dioscorea villosa)*, which is reported to be good for painful arthritis, since it has actions similar to those of cortisone.
- St.-John's-wort *(Hypericum perforatum)*, which eases pain and speeds healing, especially the healing of damaged nerves.

• Feverfew *(Tanacetum parthenium)*, which is an especially good herb for the type of arthritis or rheumatism in which muscle pain is also involved.

Allopathic Drugs

In my opinion, and the opinions of other alternative-medicine practitioners who have studied the literature on allopathic medicines, the most common Western drugs used for inflammation and pain — steroids, salicylates (aspirin and aspirin substitutes), and nonsteroidal anti-inflammatory drugs (NSAIDs) — are definitely *contraindicated* for treating arthritis. Long-term use (anything more than a couple of weeks) of any of these drugs causes nasty side effects, such as stomach ulcers and liver and kidney problems. In addition, these agents actually inhibit the healing of joint surfaces, tendons, and ligaments. What's even worse, many of them also promote degeneration of the joint-surface cartilage — the very process we are trying to prevent.

Step 6: Herbs for Arthritis

Herbs are helpful additions to the other alternative-medicine treatments. The key is to match the herbal prescription to the critter and her particular form of arthritis. This is not always an easy task; references cite more than a hundred herbs that have been effective for someone-or-other's arthritis, and no one herb will work for all cases of the disease.

Some of my favorite herbs for arthritis are:

Turmeric *(Curcuma longa)*, an anti-inflammatory herb that has been effectively used as a specific for arthritis. Turmeric is one of the ingredients of curry, and I've found that many cats like the taste of this herb.

Frankincense *(Boswellia* spp.), another herb traditionally used for arthritis. Like turmeric, frankincense is a popular arthritis treatment in Ayurvedic medicine.

Devil's claw *(Harpagophytum procumbens)*, an herb from South Africa. It is a potent anti-inflammatory and a specific for treating arthritis and rheumatism.

Alfalfa *(Medicago sativa)* and **yucca root** *(Yucca* spp.), herbs that have traditionally been used to treat arthritis. Alfalfa may be one of the best of the traditional herbal treatments, with 10 percent of humans treated responding well and others gaining partial relief. The best part of these two herbs is that they can be grown in your own backyard.

Burdock *(Arctium lappa)*, which is good for rheumatic pains, especially if skin lesions are also present.

For arthritis herbs, I prefer to sprinkle them over the cat's dinner. This type of administration gives your cat the benefit of

Alfalfa

all of the herb's "inner medicines" as well as offering more safety than herbal extractions (tinctures), which may contain potentially toxic concentrations of one biochemical. However, some of the specific arthritic herbs, such as devil's claw, frankincense, and turmeric, may have an increased medicinal action when they are used in the concentrated doses found in tinctures or capsules/tablets. In these cases, I use the human dose listed on the product label, adjusted to the cat's size.

Be Patient

Let me repeat my original word of caution: Do not expect significant results from an alternative treatment for at least 60 to 90 days. Assume that you may need to try several supplements or herbs until you find the proper mix for your pet. And resign yourself to the fact that your cat will most likely need those special supplements and herbs for the rest of his life. Remember that you've chosen the wisest and safest treatment possible.

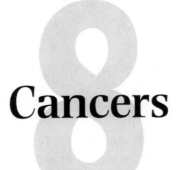

Cancers

I love the media-generated image of one of my heroes, John Wayne, limping out to the front steps of the hospital where he'd just survived cancer therapy, and growling in his wonderful bull-dog-raspy voice: "Well, boys, I've just whupped the Big C."

That's the spirit I want all my cancer clients to have: "Well boys, I know my cat can whup the Big C. And, he will do it with a John Wayne swagger of confidence." You see, I know full well that a positive mental attitude is a proven cancer antidote. I believe in miracles, and I think it helps when my clients do also. But, because I'm a midwestern country boy with an overload of pragmatism, I don't want any of my clients to think I have discovered *the* miracle cure for anything. And Lord knows, as I write this, I'm at least a chapter or two away from discovering the cure for cancer.

UNDERSTANDING CANCER

When I am presented with a cat that has cancer — any cancer — I have a few visuals I think are helpful. I visualize the cancer cells as a group of rebellious teammates that have decided to play ball their own way, without regard for the rules of the game or for the benefit of the other members of the team (the other cells of the body). These anti-team members, if allowed to grow in size and number, will eventually steal enough from the rest of the team (the rest of the body) to kill it. It's my job as a holistic veterinarian to rein in the rebellious cells and convince them that they should once again function as good team members.

Another way I look at cancer is as a lack of internal balance. A healthily functioning body works in balance: All organ systems perform their duties harmoniously and as needed. When healthy, the animal's body, mind, heart, and spirit are also in a natural state of balance. Cancer is the ultimate disease of imbalance. When cancer appears, something within the intricate homeostatic mechanisms of the cat's body has gone totally awry. If we are to "whup the Big C," we need to help your cat's body regain its state of natural homeostasis. When this happens, all the organ systems will be functioning properly, and the body, mind, heart, and spirit will once again be balanced.

Where Do Herbs Fit In?

I don't expect herbs to perform anticancer miracles. I think the best way to use them in cancer patients is as organ system balancers — improving the function of organs under attack by cancer cells and enhancing overall body mechanisms to give the cat's body its best chance to recover. Then, I always hope that one of the herbs I select will be the one that particular patient needs, along with the other therapies I am recommending, to "whup the Big C."

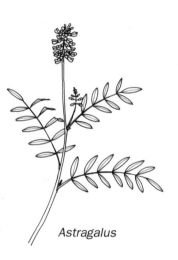
Astragalus

ANTICANCER PROTOCOL

My final piece of wisdom on cancer therapy is that the best long-term results I have seen have come when we go beyond thinking in terms of a single magic formula for a cure and develop a complete program of holistic health. I use my 10-step protocol (see chapter 2) because it gives me a basis for a complete system of holistic care. In addition to that, my special anticancer protocol includes the following steps:

1. Develop a positive belief system.
2. Eliminate as many potential causes of cancer as possible.
3. Add nutritional and supplemental support.

4. Use classical homeopathy.
5. Incorporate herbs that enhance organ function (and possibly act as an anticancer therapy).

Step 1: Develop a Positive Belief System

Use your best John Wayne swagger to create and maintain a positive attitude. Prayer, whatever your religious affiliation, has been proven to help in the healing process. Don't underestimate the power of this step.

Step 2: Eliminate All Potential Causes of Cancer

Go through your cat's entire environment. Modify it so that she avoids contact with pesticides, herbicides, airborne pollutants, and toxic household chemicals in the carpets, in the furniture, under the sink, and in the garage. Give her filtered water and serve it and her food in nonplastic (ceramic or glass) dishes.

Step 3: Add Nutritional and Supplemental Support

Perhaps the most effective component of any cancer cure is to put your cat on a good diet. Home-cooked organic foods are best. There are commercially available health foods that do not contain preservatives, and they are made from mostly organic (or hormone-, antibiotic-, pesticide-, and herbicide-free), high-quality foods.

Supplements are an excellent addition to a quality diet. Use therapeutic levels of antioxidants — vitamins A and C and the culinary herbs — and add extra levels of zinc, selenium, and omega-3 fatty acids (flaxseeds).

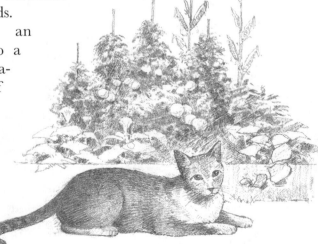

Good nutrition and helpful supplements are keys to successful cancer treatment.

Miracles

I believe in miracles, I really do. I have to; by using alternative medicines, I see miracles almost every day. But I tell all my clients: I do not know of any alternative treatment, herbal or otherwise, that will work for all cancers, every time. Whenever I think I have found an herb that is always (or even most of the time) effective, the very next patient proves me and my chosen herb wrong.

I cringe whenever I hear of someone who claims to have found a cancer cure. I call such people Cancer Charlatans. They are often well-meaning folks who have seen a cancer case (or several) respond favorably to some magic formula, but they have not tried their magic on enough patients to know that it will not work on every patient. Some are simply money grubbers with a financial interest in some form of foo-foo dust they can sell to clients who are desperate for a cure.

I consider many of the proponents of Western medicine's approach to cancer therapy to be Cancer Charlatans, too. I think that when they talk to clients, they generally tend to overestimate the percentage of cancer cases that are cured long-term by surgery, chemotherapy, or radiation therapy. But what's even worse, they often grossly underestimate the likelihood of severe adverse side effects from their methods.

I tell all my cancer clients to hope and pray for a miracle. I am also comfortable telling them that many, but not all, animals have a fair to good response to alternative therapies. Most of my patients even seem to enjoy a decent quality of life while they are undergoing therapy — this is in direct contrast to those undergoing chemo and radiation therapies. I advise my clients that alternative therapies are typically slow — often taking several months before they begin to show a positive response. Finally, I am the first to admit that some cases have not responded to anything I've tried, and unfortunately, I have never been able to predict which ones will respond and which ones will not.

Step 4: Use Classical Homeopathy

I have not found any medicine as powerful as classical home-opathy . . . when it works. With classical homeopathy you need to find the one remedy that best connects with the patient's totality of symptoms, and finding this one remedy can be a challenge. (I will occasionally use acupuncture for some cancers, but homeopathy is most often my alternative treatment of choice.) Consult a holistic vet for more information.

Step 5: Incorporate Herbs to Enhance Organ Function

When the organ systems are balanced, the body is better able to fight cancer. The major herbs I use are those that enhance organ system function, aiding the organs that are under attack by the cancer cells. For more information on herbs for the different body systems, refer to the rest of the chapters in Part 2.

HELPFUL HERBS

There are many herbs that have been successfully used to treat various cancers, and I have tried most of them at one time or another. Sometimes they work, sometimes not — it seems to be an entirely individual matter. But because many plants also enhance organ system function, they are well worth trying.

Aloe (Aloe vera)

The juice of the leaves of aloe has been used internally to stop the spread (metastases) of tumors, though it apparently does not affect the main tumor growth.

Aloe

Astragalus (Astragalus membranaceus)

In addition to enhancing the immune system, astragalus contains an alkaloid (swainsonine) that inhibits the spread of melanoma, a skin cancer.

Chaparral (Larrea *spp.*)

This herb contains a bioactive ingredient (nordihydroguaiaretic acid or NDGA) that has shown antitumor activity in the mammary glands of rats. NDGA has also been used as a commercial antioxidant in fats and oils, and chaparral contains flavones.

Echinacea (Echinacea *spp.*)

This important herb doesn't treat the cancer itself, but it has an indirect cancer prevention action by balancing the immune system. As we've seen, the health of the immune system is key to the health of the body as a whole.

Garlic (Allium sativum)

This common herb incorporates many sulfur-containing compounds, which are helpful in enhancing the immune system. One of these compounds, diallyl sulfide, has been shown to inhibit chemically caused cancers of the stomach and lungs in mice. Research also shows that garlic shortens the time it takes tumor cells to double and stimulates the growth of beneficial cells. Consumption of the plant is associated with reduced deaths from cancer. However, recent research has indicated that garlic causes Heinz body anemia in animals, especially in cats, so I am very cautious with its use.

Siberian Ginseng (Eleutherococcus senticosus)

Not to be confused with *Panax* ginseng, Siberian ginseng has been linked to inhibited tumor growth in rats. It is also a potent enhancer of the immune system.

Green Tea (Camellia sinensis)

One of those herbs that seems to have unlimited potential, green tea is a stimulant and immune-system booster. It's also an antioxidant, an astringent, and has been shown to combat some stomach and skin cancers.

Pau d'Arco (Tabebuia *spp.*)

A tea made from the inner bark of this tree, which is found in South America, has been reported to have antitumor activity.

The Best of the Rest

There are many, many herbs that have been used traditionally to treat cancers, and it is often difficult (or impossible) to separate the glowing claims from the facts. I look at it this way: If the herb has otherwise beneficial activities, why not use it in the hope that it may be successful for treating a particular cancer? If, on the other hand, the herb has many negative side effects, then I am much more cautious. My primary safe-to-use herbs include:

- Goldenseal *(Hydrastis canadensis)*
- Burdock *(Arctium lappa)*
- Red clover *(Trifolium pratense)*
- Bloodroot *(Sanguinaria canadensis)*
- Cat's claw *(Uncaria tomentosa)*
- Noni juice *(Morinda citrifolia)*

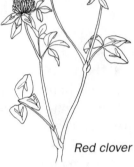
Red clover

Essiac

Essiac is an herbal cancer therapy developed by a Canadian nurse, Renee Caisse. (Essiac is Caisse spelled backwards.) This treatment is controversial because researchers have not been able to prove that it has any antitumor activities. However, thousands of people have claimed that it effectively treated their cancers, and I have had some clients who claim to have had great success with it in their cats. Essiac contains burdock root, Indian rhubarb *(Rheum palmatum),* sorrel *(Rumex acetosa),* and slippery elm *(Ulmus fulva).*

The Cardiovascular System

The cardiovascular system is an incredible, almost magical, mechanical wonder. Think about it. The system's workhorse is a pump that pulsates day and night throughout a cat's lifetime, beating consistently at the rate of about 110 to 140 beats per minute. This pump would fit into a shot glass, but it is capable of sending gallons of blood through a miles-long labyrinth of outbound arteries and returning veins.

But the heart and its supporting network of vessels are more than a mere organ. In many cultures the heart also holds a mysterious, almost mystical quality. In our culture, for example, we often think of the heart in mythological terms: We believe our hearts when they tell us we have fallen in love. We open our hearts to those we trust. And we are heartbroken when someone close to us dies.

In Chinese medicine the heart is seen as the center of consciousness, feelings, and thoughts. It houses the spirit of shen; the

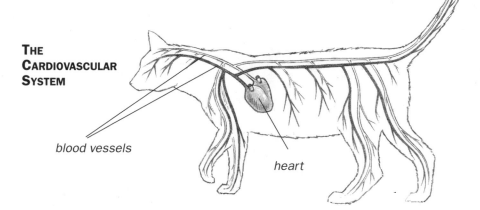

THE CARDIOVASCULAR SYSTEM

blood vessels

heart

Chinese written character for shen can be translated as spirit, soul, God, godly, and effectiveness. The meaning of this principle is touched upon when one says that an animal has spirit. Cats with mental imbalances of hysteria, such as an animal that panics and runs away, spits or hisses at the least little thing, meows incessantly, or unaccountably roams and paces, have a problem with heart shen. Some seizure patterns are also attributable to heart imbalances.

DISEASES OF THE CARDIOVASCULAR SYSTEM

While the heart may be an almost unbelievably powerful muscular organ, it can also develop problems. Symptoms that could indicate heart disease in cats include:

- Difficulty breathing
- Coughing
- General weakness
- Fainting

When the veterinarian suspects heart disease she places her stethoscope over the cat's chest and listens for any one of a cacophony of irregular sounds: heart murmurs, slowed or quickened heart rate, fibrillation, premature beats, lung congestion — any of these may indicate that something is amiss within the system. Further tests might include electrocardiography, X rays, ultrasound evaluation, blood chemistry analysis, and heartworm tests.

What Are the Causes?

Cardiovascular disease has many causes— infectious, mechanical, nutritional, hormonal, and parasitic. Here are some of the most common:

- **Bacterial infections** often find residence in the heart's valves, causing initial mechanical obstruction with possible latent damage to the valves themselves.
- **Heartworms** can mechanically block the valves, and if enough are present they can clog an entire heart chamber.
- **Hormones,** especially thyroid hormones, affect heart function; hyperthyroid cats may have a heart rate that is fast and powerful enough to be seen and felt through the chest wall.

• **Nutritional deficiencies,** such as a lack of vitamin E or selenium, may damage heart muscles. Taurine deficiency, which is seen in cats that are not on meat diets, is especially dangerous. (See the box below for more information.)

Interestingly, the primary causes of cardiovascular disease in humans, arterial cholesterol deposits and arteriosclerosis, are only very rare problems in cats — if they occur at all. Specific therapy for any cardiovascular disease will, of course, depend on the diagnosis, but herbal medicines can be used to aid whatever therapy is used.

At least 15 percent of cases of heart disease in cats are due to congenital causes — birth defects of the valves, vessels, and nerves that regulate the heart's ability to pulse naturally. Herbs offer the perfect mild, supportive care without appreciable adverse side effects. In fact, I've found the holistic/herbal approach to congenital abnormalities to be simpler and just as effective, if not more effective, than Western medicine's bell-and-whistle drugs.

THE DANGERS OF TAURINE DEFICIENCY

Hypertrophic cardiomyopathy, an enlargement of the left ventricle of the heart, may be the biggest cause of heart problems in cats. This disease can be caused by taurine deficiency.

Taurine is an essential amino acid that is made from the metabolism of the sulfur amino acids methionine and cysteine. Cats do not synthesize taurine well, so it must be supplied in the diet. The best source of taurine is meats. This means that cats are obligate carnivores; they have to eat meat to remain healthy.

After several years of a taurine-deficient diet, a cat will develop an enlarged heart. As the heart becomes larger and less efficient as a pump, edema of the lungs, weakness, lethargy, and blood clots often result. Treatment includes diuretics, cardiac-helper herbs, and taurine supplements.

A Holistic Treatment Plan

My holistic regimen for helping the cardiovascular system's diseases hinges on a four-pronged approach:

1. Herbs specific for the heart
2. Diuretics. Because a diseased heart cannot pump blood properly, many patients with cardiac disease have concurrent congestion of the lungs. Diuretics help eliminate the excess fluids
3. Other herbs that are supportive for the cardiovascular system
4. Nutritional supplements

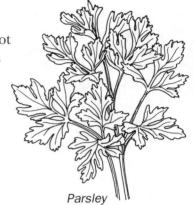

Parsley

SPECIFIC HERBS

Heart-specific herbs work in several ways, depending on the herb. They may:

- Have a normalizing effect on cardiac output, either depressing or stimulating it, depending on need
- Dilate coronary vessels, improving blood supply to the heart
- Have an overall anabolic effect on metabolism, creating a decrease in oxygen consumption and energy use
- Normalize cardiac rhythm
- Inhibit platelet aggregation (blood clotting)

Hawthorn (Crataegus laevigata)

This plant is quite simply the best heart medicine available. It acts as a cardiac tonic, normalizing the heart's activity by either depressing or stimulating its action (depending on the need). Therefore, hawthorn is good for heart failure or weakness, for heart palpitations, and as a general tonic for the circulatory system.

Hawthorn works by dilating vessels, including coronary arteries, thus enhancing the metabolic processes in the heart muscles and improving blood supply to the heart and the rest of the body. It has an overall anabolic effect on metabolism; the herb creates a decrease in oxygen consumption and energy use. This means that when the heart is under stress, hawthorn helps improve its capacity for work. Hawthorn also abolishes some types of rhythmic disturbances. In addition, it has a mild diuretic effect and has been used traditionally as an anti-inflammatory.

Hawthorn, like most herbs, does not work quite as fast as some allopathic drugs, so it is not to be used for emergencies, such as fibrillation. However, hawthorn has a synergistic effect with the drug digitalis; when used in combination, the necessary digitalis dose may be reduced to about half of that normally prescribed. Compared with digitalis, hawthorn is safer and milder in activity — there is not a cumulative effect (a buildup that increases the positive and negative effects of the medicine) with hawthorn, and hawthorn may actually decrease some of the adverse side effects of digitalis.

Almost no toxicities have been reported with hawthorn, but you should still check with a qualified herbalist before you combine hawthorn with other cardiac drugs.

Motherwort (Leonurus cardiaca)

This cardiac tonic is also used as a sedative and a female-hormone normalizer. It is an excellent tonic for the heart, strengthening the muscle without making it strain. Motherwort is especially good for conditions where the heart rate is increased because of anxiety and tension. The herb works by improving metabolism of heart muscles, reducing heart rate, increasing coronary perfusion (blood flow to the heart through the coronary arteries), and inhibiting platelet aggregation (clot formation).

For the female cat, motherwort can be used to help prepare the uterus for pregnancy. During delivery, the herb can be used to promote contractions. Since motherwort promotes uterine contractions, it should not be used during the midphases of pregnancy.

Motherwort is generally free of toxicities, but some people may develop contact dermatitis from handling it.

Motherwort

DIURETIC HERBS

An animal with a heart that is not working up to snuff often has an accumulation of fluids throughout the body (referred to as edema or ascites). These excess fluids can be especially evident in the lungs, where they can be heard with a stethoscope as fluid sounds (or moist rales). The lung-accumulated fluids often cause persistent coughing. Diuretic herbs make the animal urinate more frequently, helping to eliminate these excess fluids.

Dandelion (Taraxacum officinale)

Dandelion root is my favorite herbal diuretic. It is a potent one, but it is also liver supportive. Many diuretics in Western medicine deplete potassium, and this has an adverse effect on all muscles, especially heart muscles. Dandelion is a rich source of potassium, resupplying the amount lost in the urine.

For the great majority of cardiovascular problems I see in cats, I recommend herbal medicines along with nutritional supplements and moderate exercise. In my opinion, these three therapies are the treatments of choice.

Other Diuretics

Other diuretics that you may want to consider include:

- Cleavers *(Galium aparine)*, which is also good for lymphatic swellings, dry skin, and urinary tract infections
- Motherwort, a good herb for anxiety and female reproductive problems
- Parsley *(Petroselinum crispum)*, a hypotensive that is also beneficial for liver and gallbladder problems
- Yarrow *(Achillea millefolium)*, which is often used for fevers, infections, and liver and gallbladder problems

SUPPORTIVE HERBS

While the supportive herbs may not have a specific action on the heart, they are important for other reasons. For example, cayenne is a general tonic and it has systemic stimulative effects.

Cayenne (Capsicum spp.)

This herb can be extremely helpful for the cardiac patient because of its systemic stimulant effects. It is a general tonic, specific for the circulatory and digestive systems. Cayenne regulates blood flow, equalizing and strengthening the heart, arteries, capillaries, and nerves. Since it is a general stimulant, I also consider it good for helping deliver other herbs and nutrients to all parts of the body.

Ginger (Zingiber officinale)

Well known as an aid for digestive problems, ginger is also used as a stimulant for peripheral circulation. In addition, ginger acts as a diaphoretic, promoting perspiration. Unlike humans, cats can generate only small amounts of skin sweat. When a cat needs to cool down, he pants and may drool. Some cats sweat profusely through their paws when they are nervous or overheated. It's difficult to say how efficient herbal diaphoretics are for cats, but since toxins can be removed via sweating, any amount of increased sweat may be helpful.

Ginseng (Panax spp.)

This is a good example of an herb with bidirectional effects: Some of its compounds increase heart rate if needed; other compounds decrease heart rate when indicated. Ginseng enhances physical vitality and can be especially helpful for the older cat that is weak or exhausted, or for the depressed cat.

NUTRITIONAL SUPPLEMENTS

If your cat has cardiovascular problems, he should be on a low-sodium diet. Include a moderate amount of daily exercise, without undue stress or the strain of overexertion. Nutritional supplements can also be helpful. Consider:

- Vitamins A, B_6, C, and E; folic acid; and carnitine; these are antioxidants and/or blood thinners.
- The minerals selenium (deficiencies are linked to heart disease) and magnesium (which improves heart function).
- Fatty acids, which can be supplied through flaxseed oil (omega-3 fatty acids) or evening primrose or borage oil (primarily omega-6 fatty acids); these essential fatty acids protect heart muscle cells.

Whether or not to use one of the above depends on each individual case. But the one supplement I almost always prescribe for heart problems is coenzyme Q_{10}, a potent antioxidant that improves heart muscle oxygenation and seems to protect against heart attacks.

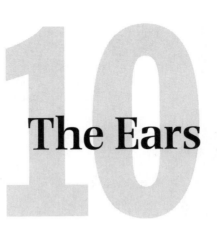

The Ears

Cats do not have nearly the number or intensity of ear problems that dogs exhibit. Perhaps it's because those little upright ears are not as safe a haven for infections as are the loppy, floppy ears of dogs. Most feline ear problems are related to ear mites.

Cats sometimes contract otitis externa, or external ear infection. This condition is caused by a wide variety of microorganisms — bacteria, fungi, and yeasts. It can also be the result of other primary causes, such as hypersensitivity diseases, foreign bodies, hypothyroidism, autoimmune diseases, disorders of the skin that involve its protective keratin layer, other systemic diseases, parasites, conformation of the ear and ear canal, and even the use of inappropriate treatments or irritating cleansers in the ear. In people, food allergies and secondary cigarette smoke have been linked to ear infections. But ear mites, *Otodectes cyanotis,* are a very common occurrence in cats, especially kittens. In fact, more than 50 percent of ear infections in cats are due to mites.

If your cat has an external ear infection, she may shake her head, cry, and scratch the affected ear(s). The ear(s) may feel hot and show evidence of scratching and irritation. Gently swabbing the ear canal with a large chunk of cotton may reveal a gooey brown to black discharge. (Ear mites often produce a dark black, crusty type of exudate.)

Otitis externa will respond to herbal and other alternative treatments. However, otitis media and otitis interna — infections of the middle and inner ear, respectively — are problems for your veterinarian only. Be sure to get an accurate diagnosis before you begin home treatment on your own.

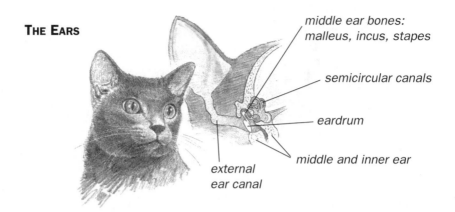

THE EARS

middle ear bones: malleus, incus, stapes

semicircular canals

eardrum

middle and inner ear

external ear canal

HOW TO TREAT IT

In Western medicine treatment, the ear canal is flushed and cleaned. Then various antibiotic or combined antibiotic/steroid preparations are used. For ear mites most Western-trained vets would use a remedy specifically aimed at killing the mites, applying the drug several times over the course of a few weeks.

Mullein Otic Mix

USE FOR: EXTERNAL EAR INFECTIONS

I like mullein *(Verbascum thaspus)* as a home-brew ear medicine because it's so easy to come by: Simply scour the local fields in late summer and collect the flowering spikes.

Mullein flowers or cob
Olive oil
Garlic

1. You can take the time to pick off the mullein flowers (a tedious process at best), or you can simply cut up the entire cob, flowers and all.
2. Pack the flowers or cob pieces loosely in a glass jar. Cover them with olive oil. For increased antibiotic effectiveness, add a clove or two of garlic per pint of oil.
3. Let the mixture sit for 2 to 3 weeks. Strain and rebottle the liquid.
4. To use, apply several drops of the oil, warmed to body or room temperature, into the ear canal. When stored in the refrigerator, the oil will last for several months.

In my opinion, alternative medicine is much better suited to treating ear infections. Herbs are a primary line of defense and my first treatment choice. In addition, chiropractic care of the neck may be helpful, and acupuncture and homeopathy are often highly effective.

In this chapter I present my own special ear treatment protocol.

Step 1: Get an Accurate Diagnosis

You must see your veterinarian for this step. First, I rule out all possible secondary causes of ear trouble (see page 73). Then I visually examine the canal with an otoscope and take a swab to identify the primary bugs involved and the severity of the disease. I use this information to decide on the overall treatment regimen.

Step 2: Employ Chiropractic

Many of the chronic ear infections I see also have cervical (neck) subluxations, or partial dislocations. Is this problem the cause or effect of the ear disease? I don't know, but adjusting the upper cervical vertebrae makes sense to me. I've seen some dramatic cures for ear conditions with chiropractic and mild herbs alone.

Step 3: Use a Vinegar Solution

If the ears are relatively clean, a mild 1:1 mix of any type of vinegar and water, applied into the ear canal, may be sufficient. You may also use an occasional herbal preparation (see page 78 for specific suggestions) instead. How often you use the vinegar/water or herbal solution depends on the individual case; it ranges from once daily for a few weeks to once a week or so for several months, then once every month or so thereafter.

ADMINISTERING EAR MEDICATION

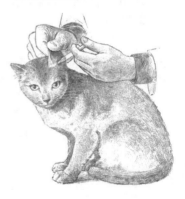

The key to giving ear meds is to get plenty of the liquid down into the ear canal. Hold the ear up and away from the cat's head, and pour (or squirt from a dropper) several drops of medicine into the canal.

Massage gently below the ear. Wipe off the excess fluid and any crud that has worked its way up from below.

Note: A key to curing ear infections is getting the herbal mixture into contact with the offending bugs. Have your veterinarian show you how to properly apply vinegar or herbal solutions so that they reach deep into the ear canal. And remember: It is much easier to prevent an infection than it is to cure it. I recommend using a mild herbal ear remedy once a month or so throughout your cat's lifetime.

Step 4: Add Herbs

For obviously infected cases I use a variety of herbal remedies. I consider these remedies as a three-pronged approach:

1. When applied topically in the ear canal, the herbs bring the ear's flora back into balance.
2. When used topically and internally (as a tea, tincture, or capsules/tablets), the plants enhance the immune system and thwart microorganism overgrowth.
3. When used topically or internally, the herbs relieve pain and inflammation (topical application is usually more effective).

Once again, how often and for how long you use the herbal mixtures depends on the individual case — from once or twice daily for a few weeks to once a week or so for several months.

Step 5: Other Alternative Treatments

For severe or chronic cases of otitis, I add either homeopathic remedies or acupuncture. It's not often that I recommend any one product, but I have found Halo's Natural Herbal Ear Wash™ very effective for otitis — whether mild or severe, acute or chronic. This product contains chamomile extract, sage oil, clove oil, horehound extract, southernwood extract, calendula extract, pennyroyal oil, and St.-John's-wort oil in a witch hazel base. It seems to ease the pain in most cases, evaporates readily in the canal (leaving no oily mess), smells good, *and* is effective. This is my starter formula for all ear problems, and I use it on my own critters as well as for my human family's earaches. It is available in many health food stores, in pet stores, or by calling (800) 426-4256.

ESPECIALLY FOR EAR MITES

While ear mites can be annoying to both owner and cat, they are relatively easy to clear up — if we are persistent and give several treatments over the course of 3 weeks. Almost any natural oil-based ear medication, even one that does not directly kill the mites, will ultimately drown them. (The oil covers the mites' breathing pores, eventually suffocating them.)

Ear mites are highly contagious, even though they are usually only found in younger animals, so you will want to treat all of the animals in the household. Don't forget to treat any dogs that are in contact with the infested kitties; dogs are also susceptible to the mites. And even if only one ear appears infected, treat both ears. The mites readily migrate over an animal's head, from one ear to the other.

I usually recommend an oil-based herbal treatment every day for about a week, then every second or third day for 2 more weeks. You need to treat your cat for 3 weeks in order to catch the mite eggs as they hatch. (Mites have a life cycle of about 3 weeks.)

TAKING THE HERBAL APPROACH

The good news is that herbal remedies are effective against fungal and yeast as well as bacterial infections. So, herbal ear infection remedies won't allow the yeast overgrowth common with antibiotic use. What's more, several of the following herbs (chamomile, mullein flowers, witch hazel) relieve the pain, inflammation, and irritation common with ear problems. So, when using herbs, you almost never need to resort to ear medications that contain those nasty steroids.

On the other hand, herbal remedies are not the magic formula for all ear infections. Remember that herbs tend to act slowly. You and your cat may not be able to put up with the head-shaking, ear-scratching, caterwauling routine while the infection heals. But it's been my experience that herbal remedies actually work nearly as fast as other veterinary drugs, and whatever we lose in quickness of response we gain back with a more completely healed ear.

Finally, not all ear infections respond to herbal remedies. In fact, I find the really chronic cases to be some of the most challenging problems I face in my alternative practice. Whenever I am presented with a chronic ear infection, I always, *always* bring out the big guns — chiropractic and either homeopathy or acupuncture — in addition to herbs.

The following is a list of my favorite herbs for otitis. Many of these are available commercially, usually as a mixture of several herbs prepared in tinctures or herbal oils. Look for them in health food stores or better pet stores. For an easy-to-make-at-home preparation for mild infections, see page 74.

Chamomile (Anthemus nobilis; Matricaria recutita)

This herb is useful when applied both internally and topically into the ear canal. Chamomile's relaxing, anti-inflammatory, analgesic, sedative, and antiseptic qualities are the perfect combination for sore, infected ears. And the herb has a powerful ability to ease your cat and help her sleep through the pain while also fighting the infection and inflammation.

St.-John's-Wort (Hypericum perforatum)

Whether used internally or externally, St.-John's-wort has antibiotic properties. It's also a wonderful herb to calm the beast made savage by the irritation of infection.

Calendula (Calendula officinalis)

Calendula, which is sometimes called pot marigold (but is not the same plant as the ornamental marigold you might have on your porch), has amazing healing abilities. It is one of the best herbs for treating local skin infections and external ear problems. Used either internally or externally, it is a potent antifungal.

Mullein (Verbascum thapsus)

An extract of mullein made in an olive oil base (see recipe on page 74) is perhaps the best single remedy I've found for soothing and healing inflamed surfaces. For otitis, place several drops of the solution deep into the ear canal.

Mullein

Other Herbs

Some other herbs are also good for treating ear infections:

- Garlic *(Allium sativum)* is often added to herbal otic mixtures for its antibiotic properties.
- Witch hazel *(Hamamelis virginiana)* is an excellent astringent, decreasing swelling in the ear canal and thus easing pain.
- Echinacea (*Echinacea* spp.) and Oregon grape root (*Mahonia* spp.) — when used internally in a combination tea, tincture, or capsule/tablet — balance the immune system and help counterattack microbes from the inside out.

Homeopathy and Acupuncture for Otitis Externa

I've found both acupuncture and homeopathy to be excellent for otitis externa, and I often resort to one or the other (in addition to herbs and chiropractic) for a severe or chronic infection. However, these are not methods for the neophyte.

It usually takes three to five initial acupuncture treatments before we see good results, and for lasting effects we may need to repeat the treatments periodically. Furthermore, specific acupuncture application around the ear is tricky (especially on a squirming cat), and a complete acupuncture treatment will always include other sites involved with immune function, organ systems related to the ear, chi, and yin-yang balance.

For home application, acu*pressure* can be very helpful. Simply massage the cat's legs, fore and hind, inside and out, from the hip and the shoulder to the toes. Then massage along the sides of your cat's spine from the head to the tail; do this *gently*. Finally, massage all the way around the base of your cat's ears.

When I use homeopathic remedies for any problem, I use classical homeopathy. The objective of classical homeopathy is to find the *one* remedy that matches the patient's constitution. Use that remedy appropriately and all diseases are cured, from the inside out.

The Eyes

When your cat has a problem with his eyes, it will not be too difficult to spot. The key symptom of eye disease is reddened eyes, often with a discharge that varies from clear tearing to a thicker, more mucuslike mess accumulating at the corners of the eyes. In general, the greater the amount of discharge and the thicker and more gooey it is, the more serious the problem. Your cat may also squint one or both eyes, and he may refuse to go into brightly lit areas. Sneezing is sometimes a part of the overall symptoms, as well.

Diagnosing the cause of the problem requires a veterinarian's thorough eye — and whole body — exam. Bacterial and viral infections of the eyes are common, and fungal infections also can cause problems. Herpes viral infections may indeed be the most common infectious eye condition seen in cats. Much like they do in people, allergies and air pollutants may cause your cat's eyes to redden and tear. Foreign bodies are a common finding, and since they typically hide behind the third eyelid they can be a real challenge to detect. Trauma (scratches and pokes from sharp objects) can tear and ulcerate the cornea (outer coating of the eye). We need to watch these eye injuries closely to be certain they don't ulcerate further.

You also need to think about other problems that may be reflected in the eyes. For example, many generalized diseases, such as coronavirus-induced feline infectious peritonitis (FIP), cause secondary ocular symptoms. Upper respiratory problems may make the eyes tear, and infections of the nose (rhinitis) may extend into the eyes and the sinuses surrounding them. Tumors can form in the eyes and surrounding tissues. And cataracts, whether caused by metabolic problems (diabetes, for example) or old age, will cause gradual loss of sight and possibly tearing or redness.

Most of the eye problems I see in my practice respond very well to herbal therapy. There are several herbs that can be used internally and externally to treat a variety of eye diseases.

THE EYES

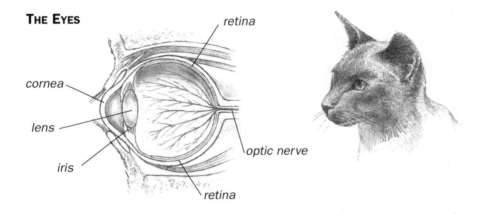

INTERNAL HERBS

Some herbs can be used internally to directly affect eye problems. Eyebright, for example, is used as an eye tonic. Ginkgo is effective against diabetic retinopathy, and bilberry has been used to protect against age- and diabetes-related changes, including macular degeneration, glaucoma, and cataracts. When used internally, these herbs also have activities that are secondarily helpful: Eyebright's anti-inflammatory, astringent, and anticatarrhal activities are beneficial for eye infections; bilberry contains several bioactive ingredients that are nourishing to the eyes; and ginkgo contains antioxidants that are helpful for the connective tissue–rich eyes.

Eyebright (Euphrasia officinalis)

An anti-inflammatory, astringent, and anticatarrhal, eyebright is an excellent remedy for easing discomfort and helping to prevent excessive tearing. This herb is rich in vitamins A and C, and it can be taken internally as a tonic for the eyes. It has also been used for centuries as an eyewash.

If the eye is infected, eyebright should be combined with anti-microbial herbs, such as echinacea (used internally) and Oregon grape root or goldenseal — both of which can be taken internally or used externally as eye drops.

Bilberry (Vaccinium myrtillus)

Rich in important nutrients that nourish the eye and enhance general visual function, bilberry also contains bioactive chemicals called anthocyanidins that help prevent damage to the structure of the eyes. It has been used to protect against age- and diabetes-related changes, including macular degeneration, glaucoma, and cataracts.

Ginkgo (Ginkgo biloba)

Ginkgo contains bioflavonoids that are helpful for connective tissue–rich organs, such as the eyes. The antioxidant properties of ginkgo protect cells and their membranes and enhance cellular metabolism and blood circulation. Recent studies indicate that ginkgo may help protect against diabetic retinopathy.

EXTERNAL HERBS (EYEWASHES)

Several herbs are used as eyewashes. Many are antimicrobial as well as anti-inflammatory and soothing. I have never seen problems when using any of these herbs as an eyewash, but some of them have caused allergic reactions in a small number of people. Use with caution, and use a very mild infusion or tea for the first time.

Selecting a Treatment

My favorite eyewash herbs are goldenseal, Oregon grape root, calendula, and chamomile. For an herb to use as an eyewash, select from this list:

- Calendula (*Calendula officinalis*), a potent vulnerary and antimicrobial
- Chamomile (*Matricaria recutita*), an excellent wound healer and anti-inflammatory
- Elder (*Sambucus nigra*), a vulnerary and anti-inflammatory
- Goldenseal (*Hydrastis canadensis*) or Oregon grape root (*Mahonia* spp.), both of which are antimicrobial and beneficial for infections involving the mucous membranes

- Meadowsweet *(Filipendula ulmaria)*, an anti-inflammatory and astringent
- Red clover *(Trifolium pratense)*, an anti-inflammatory
- Self heal *(Prunella vulgaris)*, an astringent that makes a good wash for tired or inflamed eyes

What about Commercial Products?

Many herbal eyedrop formulations for humans or animals are available commercially. Simply follow directions on these — usually a dropperful, applied to the eyes 3 or 4 times a day.

Herbal Eye Compress

Some critters are more than a handful when you're trying to get drops into their eyes. If this is the case with your cat, try a compress — a clean cloth or piece of sterile cotton soaked in herbal tea that can be applied to your cat's eyes for several minutes, several times daily. Always be very cautious when using warm liquids around your cat's eyes; the skin of the eyelid is thin and tender and can burn easily. Be sure to wash your hands both before and after treatment.

1 teaspoon fresh or dried eyewash herb of choice or a few drops of herbal extract

1 pint water

1. Simmer the herb in the water for 10 minutes. Allow the infusion to cool to a comfortable temperature.
2. Soak a clean cloth or piece of sterile cotton in the infusion. Wring it out.
3. Apply the warm, wet compress to the lid of the affected eye for 10 minutes, 4 to 6 times a day. If you use a piece of cotton, throw it away after use. If you use cloth, wash it alone in hot water with detergent and chlorine bleach (if possible) before using it again.
4. As an alternative, you can simply steep a tea bag of chamomile tea, allow it to cool to a comfortable temperature, and then apply it over the eyes several times a day.

APPLYING AN EYE COMPRESS

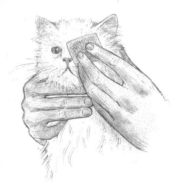

Place the warm, wet cloth or cotton directly over the lid of the affected eye.

The Gastrointestinal System

"It's not the germ, it's the soil," said Louis Pasteur. By this, Pasteur, author of the germ theory of disease and founder of microbiology, virology, and immunology, meant that the microorganism is not the major disease-causing problem; we need to look for the problem in the environment where the "bugs" grow. Nowhere is this more important than in the gastrointestinal (GI) system. I've found that nearly all the chronic diseases of a cat's stomach and gut can be corrected by paying primary attention to the GI environment. (See the Acute Intestinal Diseases box on page 86 for more information.)

We know that the billions and billions of microorganisms living in the normal gut are actually necessary to maintain a functionally healthy intestinal environment. Alter this normal flora, and you create problems. You can alter your cat's intestinal environment and flora by suddenly changing his diet — giving him foods he is

THE GASTROINTESTINAL SYSTEM

esophagus stomach large intestine

anus

small intestine

LEAKY GUT AND ALLERGIES

When yeasts are allowed to proliferate, they create a disease state that initially may be barely noticeable, characterized by headache, lethargy, malaise, sore joints, low-grade fever, and other signs of allergic response, such as skin and ear problems. The most common cause of yeast overgrowth is an inappropriate use of antibiotics or cortisone products (cortisol-producing stress may also be a cause). These medicines knock out the good-guy flora of the gut, creating the perfect environment for yeasts to grow in.

Yeasts are insidious in action, and as they continue to slowly grow and flourish, symptoms become more pronounced. Eventually the yeasts' threadlike filaments (called mycelium) penetrate the gut wall to create a condition known as leaky gut syndrome. A leaky gut allows larger than normal particles of food and food wastes into the bloodstream. These particles instigate an allergic response that settles in the gut but ultimately extends into other tissues.

Symptoms of leaky gut syndrome include persistent and chronic, often intermittent, diarrhea that is sometimes blood tinged or black from upper intestinal bleeding. Some cats also vomit. Since the gut has initiated an allergic response, your cat will often have other signs of allergies, such as arthritis, ear infections, and skin problems.

With a leaky gut, you may get temporary remission of symptoms by changing to another cat food; however, symptoms return when the cat has had enough time to develop an allergic response to the new food. As long as the yeasts are present and the gut is "leaky," your cat will eventually become allergic to any food you try, whatever its hypoallergenic claims. Fix the gut, and your cat will ultimately be able to eat almost any food.

not used to or foods too rich in proteins or sugars. These sudden changes may cause transient diarrhea or even temporary vomiting.

The most common causes of chronic gastrointestinal disease that I see are those caused by indiscriminate use of antibiotics and steroids. Use either of these medicines too often or for too long, and you set up a perfect environment for the proliferation of bad-guy bugs, mainly yeasts. (Whenever an animal is on antibiotics or steroids, I recommend concurrent addition of "good-guy" bugs, such as the lactobacillus found in unsweetened yogurt or in capsules.)

HERBS FOR ACUTE GI PROBLEMS

I've found that the holistic answer to nearly all GI diseases is to improve the GI environment (Pasteur's soil) so the natural, healthy gastrointestinal flora can take over from the bad-guy bugs causing the problem. But I've also discovered that herbal therapy is often my best choice for chronic GI problems and for most acute problems.

Slippery Elm (Ulmus rubra)

For transient diarrhea *or* constipation, I've found nothing better than slippery elm. It is a soothing nutritive demulcent that coats sensitive or inflamed mucous membranes. It is the perfect remedy for the cat with an upset belly — for example, when a change in diet causes temporary GI upset. But this herb is good for any type of stomach upset. Give ½ teaspoonful of the powdered herb (mixed with water and given as a liquid with a dropper) per 10 pounds of body weight, 4 or 5 times a day.

Slippery elm is also good for the cat with GI upset due to tension or a change in his daily routine — a cat traveling in a car, for example, or a cat made nervous by new visitors. Give the dose mentioned above several hours before your cat will be exposed to the stressful event. You can repeat the dose 4 or 5 times a day. Continue for several days if necessary.

Slippery elm

ACUTE INTESTINAL DISEASES

There are several acute GI disease problems that may be life threatening to cats. The most serious acute disease with gastrointestinal symptoms is panleukopenia (feline distemper). If this disease is not treated promptly it may prove fatal; you *must* consult your veterinarian immediately, rather than relying on herbs alone. When diarrhea contains reddish or blackish blood, or when it persists for more than a day or two, see your veterinarian.

Herbal Protocol for Chronic GI Problems

I am seeing so many cases of chronic GI disease (referred to as chronic bowel disease, inflammatory bowel syndrome, leaky gut syndrome, and other, more colorful names invented by my clients and not appropriate for a family-oriented book such as this one) that I think it will become the "designer disease" of the decade. What should we expect, after all, with all the antibiotics and steroids used in a normal Western medicine practice?

My five-step holistic program for chronic GI problems follows.

Step 1: Soothe and Heal the Gut

My favorite soothing herb is slippery elm. For chronic gut problems, I might use it for 3 or 4 weeks initially, then stop for a week, and repeat as necessary. Don't use it continuously, though; the herb is so effective as a coating agent that there is some concern that it might prevent proper absorption of nutrients with prolonged use. Another demulcent herb for coating mucous membranes is marsh mallow *(Althaea officinalis)*.

Step 2: Reduce Inflammation

Wild yam is an excellent anti-inflammatory that has been used to soothe intestinal and arthritic diseases. It also aids the function of the liver. **Licorice root** has a structure similar to that of the natural steroids of the body. It is an anti-inflammatory used especially for gastritis and peptic ulcers.

Antioxidants are important to counter the excess production of free radicals. I use high levels of vitamins A and C, combined with antioxidant herbs such as oregano, basil, and thyme. I've also recently begun using glucosamine and methylsulphonylmethane (MSM) for their anti-inflammatory activity; they are especially indicated for the animal with concurrent arthritic symptoms.

Step 3: Reestablish Normal Flora

There are two keys here:
- Increase the fiber in the gut. To achieve this, good-quality food is a must. Home cooked is best, but there are a few "gourmet" health foods on the market that have also worked well for many of us holistic vets. Fiber is easiest to supply by adding cooked oatmeal, brown rice, or cooked wheat to your cat's food. Start with about a teaspoon for every 10 pounds of cat.

- Introduce "good-guy" bugs. These include the *Lactobacillus* and *Bifidobacterium* species, and they're easiest to provide with a dollop of unsweetened yogurt atop your cat's food. Both are also available in capsules at most health food stores.

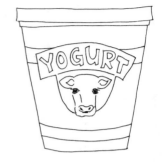

A third key for humans, but one we need not worry about for cats — unless you are one of those people who sneaks candy to Kitty under the table — is to eliminate all sugar in the diet. Yeasts love sugar.

Step 4: Diminish the Overabundance of Yeasts

For this step, I like goldenseal or Oregon grape root as anti-microbials; they are effective against both bacteria and yeasts. These herbs are also astringents (easing inflammation of the gut), and they aid liver function. Another natural remedy with specific activity against fungi and yeasts is the inner bark of the Pau d'arco tree. This remedy has also been shown to have anticancer activity.

Step 5: Enhance the Immune System

Part and parcel of chronic bowel syndrome is an immune system that has gone haywire. (Many of the animal cases of chronic bowel syndrome have a dramatic proliferation of lympho-cytic tissue surrounding the gut — direct evidence that the immune system in the area is being stimulated abnormally.) Now we'll probably never know whether this imbalance is a result of the ongoing gut disease or the other disease process started with a compromised immune system. No matter; we need to return the immune system to its normal functional state. Western medicine's answer to this is cortisone, which temporarily reduces ongoing inflammation but, in effect, shuts down the immune system for the long term. Good short-term results; perhaps disastrous long-term consequences.

In my mind it's hard to beat echinacea in balancing the immune system. Echinacea increases lymphocyte production when that is indicated and reduces production when there are already enough lymphocytes.

OTHER GASTROINTESTINAL PROBLEMS

The following gastrointestinal problems are not listed under the acute or chronic problems because they can be either acute or chronic.

Excess Gas (Flatulence)

Carminatives relax stomach muscles, increase peristalsis of the intestine, and reduce production of gas. There are plenty of aromatic herbs to choose from, one of which should give you a whiff of success. Carminative herbs include:

- Aniseed
- Cardamon
- Cayenne
- Chamomile
- Coriander
- Fennel
- Ginger
- Peppermint
- Thyme

Any of the above herbs can be the answer to your cat's aromatic activities. Use them as your cat's system seems to be asking for them: If your cat is a chronic gasser, try one or more of the listed herbs mixed in with each meal. Try different herbs and different combinations until you get the correct mix. If your cat has only occasional problems, when his diet is changed, for example, then one or more of the above herbs can be used whenever you change from one food to another.

Sluggish Digestion

Occasionally cats, especially the aged critters, will have a sluggish digestive system that simply needs to be kicked up a notch. My favorite digestion-aiding herbs include:

- Cayenne
- Dandelion root
- Ginger
- Turmeric

Since the liver is an important component of digestion, I typically would add milk thistle seeds to the herbal recipe. The same general instructions exist for these herbs as for the herbs for excess gas.

The Immune System

The immune system is my favorite body system to talk about because it gives me the chance to discuss several of the important aspects of integrating herbs into a wellness protocol for your cat's healthy body/mind.

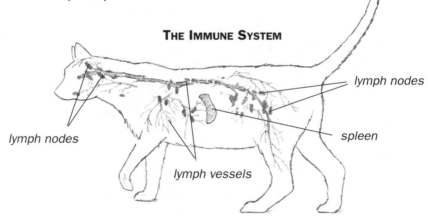

THE IMMUNE SYSTEM

lymph nodes

lymph nodes

lymph nodes

spleen

lymph vessels

WHAT IS THE IMMUNE SYSTEM?

For starters, it's important to realize that the immune system is much more than just the white blood cells (WBCs) that circulate in the blood stream. The WBCs (made up of lymphocytes and phagocytes), of course, are vital; they have the ability to recognize "foreign stuff" (everything from bacteria, viruses, and fungi to splinters, dust, and the toxic by-products of diseases and body metabolism) and then to eat (phagocytize) that stuff and remove it from the body. But WBCs are not the whole immunity package.

The Role of Proteins

Also circulating in the blood is a whole army of immune system proteins, including antibodies, the complement system, interferon, and interleukins. WBCs are not especially effective against viruses, but some of these proteins (especially interferon) are. Many of the immune-balancing herbs increase both the amount and the effectiveness of these proteins. And there's more.

How Other Organs Help

The WBCs circulating in the blood are actually a very small portion of the total number of these cells found in the body; one of the prime areas for WBCs is along the gastrointestinal tract (especially in lymphocyte-rich areas called Peyer's Patches). So herbs that help your cat's belly also aid his immune system.

The fact is, almost every organ gives a hand to your cat's immune system. The liver, for example, not only removes the toxins that decrease immune response but also is the prime manufacturing site for the immune proteins mentioned above. Add the thyroid, adrenals, spleen, and thymus to our list of immune-important organs, and it's easy to see that any time we help an organ system we also aid your cat's immunity.

We also know that most of the cells of the body have a naturally protective, surface immune capability. Lung cells, for example, produce a mucus layer that is antiseptic. Cells along the intestine produce substances (lysozymes) that are antibacterial and antiviral. Herbs that enhance individual cellular functions also indirectly enhance the immune system in general.

TREATING THE IMMUNE SYSTEM SYNERGISTICALLY

Scientific studies have shown that a stressed or depressed mind lowers immune response. In contrast, a happy cat living in a relaxed and loving environment will often have the healthiest immune system possible.

To summarize, since the immune system is actually an interconnecting whole-body network, I always use a mind-body approach whenever I prescribe herbs for *any and all* feline diseases. And since almost every disease, whether it is of the body or the mind, adversely affects the immune system, I remember to balance the immune system with appropriate herbs even as I'm treating another specific disease. So where do you begin when treating your cat's immune system?

Step 1: Prevention Is the Best Medicine

Herbs are simply the very best way to keep all of your cat's body systems at maximum performance level. I especially like the culinary herbs for this, sprinkled on the food. Try oregano, thyme, turmeric, cumin, and cayenne. Food is medicine; medicine is food.

Oregano

Step 2: Create a Healing Environment

This should be both internal and external. I don't believe any medicine is complete by itself; to be effective, *all* medicines — herbal and otherwise — need to be "planted" in a healthy environment that includes good nutrition, proper exercise, minimum stress, low levels of toxins and pollutants, and frequent doses of hands-on loving care.

Step 3: Activate All Systems

Licorice root is my favorite adaptogen, because it activates nearly all organ systems. This herb contains compounds with a chemical structure similar to that of the natural, anti-inflammatory steroids of the body. Its effects are also specific for bronchial and abdominal problems. Most pets like the taste of licorice root, making it ideal for use as a tincture or tea or as a flavoring to make other herbs more palatable.

As an alternative to the adaptogenic properties of licorice root, I may consider one of the ginsengs (especially Siberian ginseng, *Eleutherococcus senticosus)*. However, I find that because most folks don't understand all of the actions of the various ginsengs, these herbs are often abused. I generally stick to licorice root, except in special cases.

Step 4: Activate Specific Organ Systems

As an example, let's say that our diagnosis indicates liver involvement. For mild liver symptoms I include one of the liver tonics — turmeric or dandelion root — sprinkled as a dressing on the cat's food. If the liver symptoms are more severe, I might add milk thistle seed, either as an extract or sprinkled atop the food. And our old friend licorice root is also used in Chinese medicine as a liver detoxifier. Remember, by directly aiding the liver, we not only enhance detoxification (see step 5), but also indirectly affect the immune system. Your holistic vet will be able to tell you which organ systems require activation.

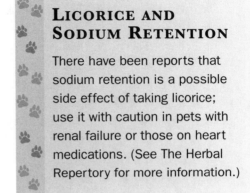

LICORICE AND SODIUM RETENTION

There have been reports that sodium retention is a possible side effect of taking licorice; use it with caution in pets with renal failure or those on heart medications. (See The Herbal Repertory for more information.)

Step 5: Detoxification

All diseases produce toxic by-products that need to be removed, including dead cellular debris, dead and dying bacteria and viruses, oxidative and other abnormal by-products from damaged cells, and chemical toxins introduced into the body from a variety of sources.

My favorite "detox" herbs are burdock root and red clover. Use them in combination, preferably on your cat's food as a tea or sprinkle. I especially like these two plants because they are well-tolerated by most cats; they counteract dry, scaly skin (a common site for immune diseases to manifest themselves); and together they may have some antitumor effects.

Step 6: Calm the Savage Beast

Nearly all the cases I see involve a pet that's a nervous wreck, for one reason or another. If the cat is anxiously pacing and crying, worrying about being sick, I'll add valerian or St.-John's-wort to his herbal formula.

If Pet's compromised immune system has given him the nighttime itchy-scratchies, I'll offer chamomile as a natural sleeping pill. I also like wild oat for its mildly calming, antidepressive effects. Sprinkle these "mind herbs" on your cat's food, giving him the chance to select the ones that appeal to his inner senses.

Step 7: Balance the Immune System

Our most notable herb for immune balancing is echinacea. Used on a periodic basis, this herb reinforces nearly all actions of immunity, including WBC production and activity and interferon and interleukin production. Echinacea also has strong wound healing activity, is anti-inflammatory, has some antitumor activity, and is mildly active against some bacteria and viruses.

There are some minor differences between *Echinacea angustifolia* and *E. purpurea* in their medicinal activity, but I use them interchangeably in practice. I use a tincture (nonalcoholic if possible) of all plant parts (leaves, flowers, and roots). Since it has such a tangy taste, for some cats you may need to camouflage it — in a favorite treat, for example.

Echinacea

If you catch an infection early, you can often stop it in its tracks with low doses of echinacea, given several times a day (every 2 to 3 hours). For prevention and general immune care I recommend a low-dose, on/off cycle; for example, 5 days on with 2 days off each week, or 3 weeks on and 1 week off. There is little, if any, scientific basis for this dosage schedule. In fact, recent clinical evidence indicates that long-term therapy may be as good, if not better. But I simply have a gut feeling that an on/off cycle is more natural.

> *Since echinacea does not simply stimulate the immune system but rather balances it, I am comfortable using it for immune diseases, such as leukemia complex, autoimmune hemolytic anemia (AIHA), immune-mediated skin and gastrointestinal problems, and immune-mediated arthritis.*

Step 8: Remove Invaders

The most common invaders are bacteria, fungi, and viruses. While herbs *can* be effective against bugs in the early stages, I try not to let any microbial infection get out of hand before I reach for a stronger medicine, even antibiotics if necessary. Echinacea, licorice root, and many of the culinary herbs (see page 92) have antimicrobial activity.

If you've caught the infection early enough, consider adding herbs such as Oregon grape root for the urinary tract; calendula for the mouth and throat; or thyme for the gastrointestinal or respiratory systems. Remember that, as a general rule, herbs are not as potent or as fast acting — nor do they have as many side effects — as antibiotics.

Keep a Holistic Perspective

Your cat's immune system is an all-encompassing, interwoven complex that is spread throughout all organ systems, including the mind. Pet's immune capability is all-important for health and disease control, no matter which disease he has. Herbs are the perfect medicine to support the immune system at all levels.

DELIVERY METHODS FOR THE IMMUNE SYSTEM

Your cat's tongue and mouth may have a vital role in his immune response. According to recent evidence, when a whole herb first enters the mouth and touches the tongue, there is a whole-body response that activates many organ systems, particularly the immune system. In fact, this initial touch of the herb may be *the* critical part of whole-body response, especially when we are talking about the immune system.

So whenever we use the oral delivery method, sprinkling whole herbs atop your cat's food, we are taking advantage of the orally induced response. In addition, the whole-herb approach gives your cat the maximum benefit of the synergistic effects of the different biochemicals within the herbs, as well as the safety factors inherent in the bidirectionality of most herbs.

The Liver

The liver is the largest organ in your cat's body, and I would argue that it is one of the most, if not *the* most, important organ of all. It is the primary site for filtering and detoxifying impurities in the blood, whether they are chemical, bacterial, or allergic. The liver processes most of your cat's food, converting nutrients and synthesizing proteins, and it manufactures bile that aids in the digestion of fats. Finally, it is a huge storage bin for several nutrients, such as glycogen (your cat's sugar source for quick energy), blood, vitamins, and iron.

Just as the liver has so many diverse functions, the symptoms related to liver dysfunction also seem unlimited. For example, many of your cat's gastrointestinal imbalances, such as diarrhea, constipation, vomiting, bloating, bad breath, excess gas, and abnormal stools, may be related to liver problems.

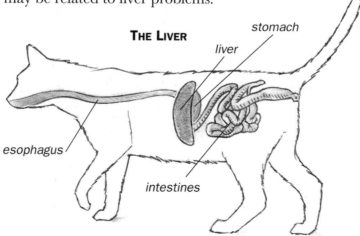

THE LIVER

stomach

liver

esophagus

intestines

Consider a liver problem whenever your cat seems to have a decrease in overall energy or a recent personality change, whether she is more anxious or more lethargic. Symptoms of the eyes (itchy, watery, swollen, red) and ears (itchy or draining ear infections) may be related to liver dysfunction, and your cat's arthritis may also be a result of liver imbalance. Finally, skin problems, especially acne and psoriasis but also rashes, dry and peeling skin, and wounds that are slow in healing, may be liver related.

Jaundice, a yellowing of the skin and the whites of the eyes, is an obvious indicator of liver dysfunction. Your vet can analyze liver function by testing for liver enzymes in the blood. But I feel that many of a cat's liver problems are already far advanced by the time jaundice appears or liver enzymes in the blood reach abnormal levels.

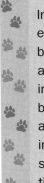

WHAT IS HEPATIC LIPIDOSIS?

In hepatic lipidosis, for as yet unknown reasons, cats accumulate excess fat in their liver cells. Contributing factors include obesity combined with several days of not eating or drinking, steroid therapy (either anabolic steroids or glucocorticoids), and a poor diet that does not include enough liver-protective vitamins. Cats with hepatic lipidosis can become extremely sick. They may be lethargic, refuse to eat, become anemic, bleed easily, and develop nervous signs related to the liver's inability to process toxins. Therapy can be extensive for cats with this syndrome, and I've found the liver herbs to be extremely helpful additions to Western medicine treatments.

HEALING PLANTS

Fortunately, a number of herbs are excellent for liver problems, and I've found that some are actually better than anything Western medicine has to offer. (If your cat has liver problems, you should also read the box about liver dysfunction on page 101.)

What's more, herbs can be used no matter what caused the liver problem, because:

- Liver-specific herbs have several modes of action that are both liver protective and liver regenerative.

- Herbs typically have a broad-based sphere of activity, enhancing the function of many organ systems that, in turn, offer support to the liver.
- Unlike many drugs that stress or damage the liver as they are metabolized, liver herbs actually enhance liver function.

In this chapter I present my favorite liver-protecting and liver-enhancing herbs. Many of these herbs can be applied as a tonic for long-term protection of the liver — not a bad idea in today's toxin-laden, stress-producing environment.

Milk Thistle (Silybum marianum)

Milk thistle benefits the liver in at least four ways. It:

Milk thistle

1. Is cholagogic, helping to increase bile flow
2. Strengthens and stabilizes cell membranes — this is especially important for cells that have been exposed to toxins
3. Acts as a potent antioxidant and slows the inflammatory response, helping prevent further damage to liver cells
4. Stimulates protein synthesis, rebuilding cells that have been damaged from any type of liver disease

While all parts of the plant are edible, the seeds are thought to contain the highest concentration of medicinal properties.

I use milk thistle to support my overall protocol for healing whenever I suspect diseases of any kind in the liver or gallbladder; this includes infectious (bacterial, viral, fungal), parasitic, toxin-produced, and oncogenic (cancerous) diseases. I've also found the herb helpful for other problems secondarily related to liver dysfunction, such as gastrointestinal upset, skin conditions, blood clotting abnormalities, dysfunctions related to the immune or hormonal systems, or hepatic lipidosis.

In addition, since milk thistle seeds are extremely safe to use and readily accepted in food by almost all pets, I recommend them as a general tonic; add a pinch of seeds to your cat's food a couple of times a week. Active ingredients of the seeds are not very soluble in water, so teas are probably not very effective. Instead, for the liver-sick cat, you should use tinctures or capsules/tablets.

Artichoke (Cynara scolymus)

Milk thistle may seem to be the cure-all for liver problems, but artichoke is yet another herb with similar, if not equal, application to liver diseases. And yes, Virginia, this is the same artichoke you relish at dinnertime. The only difference is that for liver protection we use the leaves rather than the fruits.

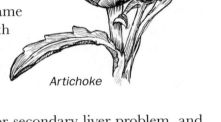

Artichoke

Artichoke is pretty much the same as milk thistle in all respects, with perhaps a bit more cholesterol-protective action (which is more important in human patients than in cats). So use artichoke whenever your cat has a primary or secondary liver problem, and consider adding some artichoke leaf sprinkles to your healthy cat's food several times a week as a good general liver tonic. Artichoke may also be combined with milk thistle — there is likely a synergistic effect when the two are used together.

Turmeric (Curcuma longa)

In my practice I usually think of turmeric and other culinary herbs as an adjunct to the medicinal herbs, but this is perhaps a mistake. After all, turmeric is an excellent cholagogue, and it exhibits liver-protective qualities similar to those of milk thistle and artichoke.

In addition to its liver-helping effects, turmeric also has:

- Anticancer properties
- Antimicrobial characteristics
- Anti-inflammatory properties
- Cardiovascular system benefits, by inhibiting platelet aggregation and interfering with intestinal cholesterol uptake
- Intestinal benefits, by decreasing gas formation.

Turmeric is a good herb to add to your cat's food as sprinkles — I am continually surprised by the number of animals that relish its taste, either alone or as a part of the mix of herbs called curry (usually a combination of turmeric, coriander, cumin, garlic, cayenne, fennel, fenugreek, anise, nutmeg, mace, cinnamon, cloves, black pepper, cardamom, ginger, and onion). Furthermore, nearly all the curry herbs are also helpful for the liver and other organ systems. Use only high-quality herbs, not the dried-out variety sold in supermarkets.

WESTERN MEDICINE AND THE LIVER

Despite the vital importance of the liver in overall health and well-being, in our culture the liver tends to be the most ignored of all of our cats' organ systems. What's more, Western medicine has few answers for liver problems. I get more questions from Western-trained veterinarians about the liver than for any other problem. Typically, their question is: "Doc, is there anything else I can do, from your holistic perspective, for this critter's liver?"

Truth be known: In veterinary school we weren't given much to work with for any disease process . . . unless the disease was related to "bugs" we could zap with antibiotics. Only through studying and working with alternative methods have holistic practitioners learned "newer" methods of liver care that include nutrition, exercise, toxin and stress elimination, body-balancing medicines (acupuncture, chiropractic, and homeopathy), and herbal therapies.

Other Herbs

I often include some other herbs in my feline patient's liver-healing preparations, especially if they are indicated because of their other qualities.

Licorice. I include this in most of my herbal formulations for its adaptogenic qualities (which help many organ systems) as well as its anti-inflammatory and antistress aspects. Because of its sweet taste, it is readily accepted by most pets. Licorice is also an antioxidant, and it helps relieve intestinal irritations, especially ulcers.

Yarrow. This mild tonic and bitter helps increase bile flow and has anti-inflammatory and antimicrobial qualities.

Dandelion. In addition to having kidney-supportive actions, dandelion also increases bile flow and has mild antimicrobial effects.

Berberine-containing herbs. Berberine compounds are effective antifungals, antibacterials, and immune enhancers (by activating macrophages). In addition, they enhance all normal digestive secretions. This category of herbs includes barberry (*Berberis* spp.) and Oregon grape root (*Mahonia* spp.).

A Protocol for Liver Dysfunction

Whenever I suspect liver problems, I use a five-step liver-healing and liver-protective protocol:

1. Decrease your pet's exposure to any toxins or agents, microbial or otherwise; these compromise liver function.
2. Provide food that has high nutritive value, low fat content, and no sweeteners, synthetic preservatives, food colorings, or artificial flavorings.
3. Since the gut often creates stress for the liver, get the gut back to normal function by resupplying beneficial organisms (lactobacilli and other normal gut flora) in the food. One teaspoon to several tablespoons (depending on the size of the cat) of unsweetened yogurt is a good addition to your cat's daily dinner. You'll also need to increase fiber intake — to decrease food transit time and provide a healthy environment for the growth of beneficial organisms — and decrease intestinal permeability via beneficial organisms and elimination of intestinal yeast. Don't forget to address intestinal yeast/candidiasis (especially if there's a history of antibiotic or cortisone use or undue stress) and intestinal parasites, if applicable.
4. Add liver-protecting agents to the diet, including B vitamins, vitamins C and E (antioxidants), lipoic acid, catechin, cysteine, and lipotrophic factors (methionine, choline, vitamin B_6, betaine, and folic acid).
5. Add liver-protective herbs.

The Nervous System

15

Some cats are calm as cucumbers. Others exhibit various degrees of nervousness, emotional stress, inner tension, anxiety, and terror. "Scaredy" cats have a variety of ways of expressing their fears: Some pace, cry, or wail, caterwauling into the night. Others run from the slightest noise or differences in their usual environs, skittering under the bed or into the closet. There are cats who express their fears and angers by eliminating in inappropriate places, such as the middle of their human's pillow. And there are cats that keep their fears and anxieties well hidden but are literally abuzz underneath their seemingly calm facade.

THE NERVOUS SYSTEM

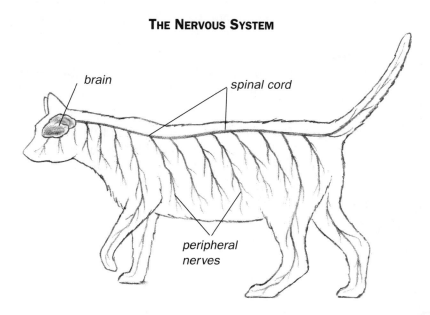

brain

spinal cord

peripheral nerves

THE KIDD'S PET SERENITY SCALE

Each of the Kidd household critters has a different ranking on the serenity scale, and each seems to have a different reason to go off the scale into pitiful fits of whining, crying, and cowering under the bed. For example, Rufus, our golden retriever, loves to ride in the car — anywhere, anytime, for as long as we want to travel. He simply watches out the window until he's tired, and then he curls up and sleeps. Quixote the cat, on the other hand, starts an ear-piercing caterwauling from the minute we open the car door until we stop at our destination — unless we give him some calming herbal help, of course.

At the first rumble of a distant thunderstorm or the sound of the first Fourth of July firecracker, Rufus is underfoot, whining and sniveling, demanding we protect him. I've never noticed the cats even lift their head from deep sleep, curled up on the couch, no matter how loud the thunder claps or how close the firecrackers.

Visitors are Rufus's cup of tea; the more the merrier. Quixote is not so impressed with strangers. He generally tries to find a sleeping place out of the way, but he will occasionally join the crowd for a short petting and purring session. Little Cat, though, is long gone when the doorbell first chimes, and you'll be lucky to see the whites of his terrified eyes from under the couch during the entire visit.

HERBS TO THE RESCUE!

I've found that herbs are the ideal calmers because they are mild in their activity and won't make your cat "crash," like more potent tranquilizers do. The activity of herbs is short lived; animals won't wake up with a "hangover." Herbal calmers are not addictive, and there is no cumulative effect — meaning that the herbs don't stay in the body and create a residue of activity from previous doses. Finally, animals do not adapt to herbal doses, meaning that you will not need to increase the herbal dose over time.

Some of the herbal calmers, particularly oat, are tonics, offering overall balance to the nervous system. Since animals have been rolling around in herbs for eons, I feel their systems are better adapted to herbs' activities, making them a much more natural approach to nervous system imbalances.

Remember to try these herbs *before* you need them; this will help you get a feel for your cat's individual reaction to them and the proper dose for each pet. Also, and perhaps most important, when Pet needs one of the herbs, take the same herb yourself. When you are calm and relaxed, your cat will follow suit. Just be sure to consult your physician or herbalist before taking a new herb, especially if you are already taking medication.

Following are my favorite herbs for the serenity-challenged cat.

Oat (Avena sativa)

This is the first herb I consider, not because it is such a powerful antidote to nervous jitters but because it is such a good general nervine and so easy to give a pet. Oat is used to strengthen and provide overall support for the nervous system. Any pet with upset nerves can benefit from a dose of oats each day or a few times a week.

Cooked oatmeal added to your cat's food will help his nerves and provide a source of fiber. You can also grow oat grass (in an indoor flowerpot during the winter). When it's a few inches tall, clip and serve, or just let your cat graze on the grass, as our critters love to do. Or you can make a tea from oat straw and soak your dog's food in it. If you choose to make a tea, be sure you use organic oat straw.

Another way to reap the benefits of this plant is to boil about a pound of shredded organic oat straw in 2 quarts of water and add it to your cat's bathwater. This makes a wonderfully calming and healing bath with high levels of skin-soothing salicylic acid. That is, it is calming *if* your cat enjoys a bath. If, on the other hand, he's like many cats, *no* bath is calming, no matter which herbs are used. If none of these delivery systems suits your fancy, oat is also available in capsule, tablet and tincture forms, or you can use the wild oat flower essence remedy.

Catnip (Nepeta cataria)

If you've ever watched a cat go gaga, excitedly rolling around in catnip leaves, this may seem like a strange choice as a calming herb. Watch Kitty after the euphoric high, however, and you'll appreciate catnip's latent calming effect. First comes the buzz (for a genetically predetermined percentage of cats — some don't feel anything), then it's time to relax.

Give your cat a healthy snifter of catnip 15 to 30 minutes before a car trip or other stressful event. Let her have her jollies, and then give her a quiet place to sleep it off. You can repeat this every couple of hours, but your cat will eventually become desensitized to repeat doses. Also, be sure to give a healthy dose of catnip at the end of the trip or grandkid's visit as a reward for putting up with the stresses of the event.

Incidentally, catnip as a tea or tincture is also calming for most animal species, especially for intestinal upsets.

Valerian (Valeriana officinalis)

Valerian: The other catnip. For many cats (again, a genetically predetermined percentage) valerian acts just like catnip. In fact, some cats are even crazier for valerian. I don't know if this is always true, but it's been my observation that many of the cats that don't respond to catnip love valerian, and vice versa. For valerian-crazed cats you'll need to keep the roots in an airtight (and claw-tight) container just to keep your cats from stealing a whiff whenever they can. There's a second reason to keep valerian locked up in an odor-tight container: The roots have the powerful, whole-room-penetrating smell of dirty socks.

Valerian is specifically used to reduce tension and anxiety, over-excitability, and hysterical states. It was the herb of choice for Londoners enduring the bombing raids during World War II, and I think of this whenever I try to match an anxious animal to the herb's calming effects. Interestingly, rats also love valerian — it is said the Pied Piper actually used a pocketful of valerian to lure the rats out of town.

Chamomile (Anthemis nobilis; Matricaria recutita)

This is another potent sedative, and it has the added advantages of calming your cat's belly and encouraging him to sleep.

Chamomile, then, is an herb to consider before the car ride over the river and through the woods to grandfather's house; it will ease the upset stomach and put your cat to sleep for the duration.

Some cats enjoy chamomile tea as much as we humans do, or you can soak a small treat with the tea. Chamomile is also available in capsules/tablets and as a tincture; see page 34 for dosage.

USING FLOWER ESSENCE REMEDIES

Bach's Rescue Remedy, Flower Essence Service's Five Flower Remedy, and other similar commercially available remedies are usually concentrated mixtures of cherry plum, clematis, impatiens, rock rose, and star of Bethlehem. Since the flower essence remedies were developed to deal with emotional disturbances, for most animals they are the premier treatments to consider for acute or severe anxiety, stress, and hysteria. They are extremely easy to give; try administering a few drops orally, dilute several drops in ½ ounce or more of drinking water, or combine a few dropperfuls with several ounces of water and spritz (with a plant mister) Pet as you travel (or as she hides under the bed).

Lavender (Lavandula angustifolia)

Lavender is a sedative that is helpful for the anxiously yowling, crying, pacing cat. Moisten your cat's food with lavender tea, or try the aromatherapy approach: Waft its fragrance into her environment. For a car trip, put a few drops of the essential oil on a cotton ball and hang it from the rearview mirror; you can also do this in the room that is your cat's favorite hiding place.

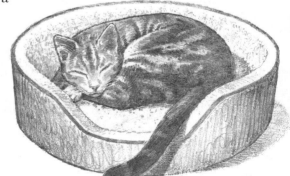

Your cat will rest easy after a dose of calming lavender.

Other Herbs

Other herbs that may be beneficial when you're considering the nervous system include:

- Skullcap, which is good for nervous tension and may have antispasmodic benefits for epileptic patients.
- St.-John's-wort, which is good for anxiety and tension or any time your cat is depressed or in need of nerve healing.
- Kava kava, an herb that will relax anxiety, tension, and restlessness, without a loss of mental sharpness

Different Herbs for Different Cats

In the Kidd family of cats, Quixote is catnip responsive — dramatically responsive. He purrs loudly and hums a song of happiness as he devours the aroma, rolling in the herb with unabated glee and rubbing sensually against anything and everything he sees. When his euphoria is over, we won't see him for hours — he's long gone to one of the bedrooms for a long siesta. But Little Cat ignores our catnip offerings, and stares at Quixote's shenanigans as if he is crazy.

Valerian is an extremely calming herb for Little Cat, after she has experienced a rather mild euphoric state brought on by the initial exposure. Quixote, on the other hand, tests the air around a fresh bit of scattered valerian, then marches out of the room in a huff.

Little Cat is not a big fan of car trips, but she calms down considerably when we put a few drops of lavender on a cotton ball hung from the rearview mirror. Quixote hates the car with a passion. We give him catnip a half-hour or so before the journey and renew the dose every 30 minutes. Even then he is still able to wake up every few minutes and loudly voice his objections to traveling.

The key here is to try a variety of calming herbs under conditions when your cat is usually stressed, until you get the right one for her individual needs.

The Reproductive System
(Neutered Cats)

For several years now I've been recommending herbal support for neutered pets. Please don't misunderstand; I am not opposed to neutering. In fact, I don't know one responsible practitioner, holistic or otherwise, who doesn't agree that the benefits of neutering far outweigh the potential problems. We are all acutely aware that excess animal population is a huge problem, and neutering is simply the best way available for us to keep the population at bay. (See The Number-One Killer of Pets in the United States on page 114 for more information.)

NEUTERING: THE OPERATION

Neutering is a major surgical procedure, performed under anesthesia and sterile conditions. Since neutering is major surgery, there is some risk — both from the surgery itself and from the potential for adverse reaction to the anesthesia. However, when done by an experienced and competent veterinarian, neutering is so low risk that we see an extremely low percentage of problems in the millions of animals neutered each year.

Female neutering, also known as spaying (from the old English *spayen,* which comes from the French word *espeer,* meaning "to cut with a sword") or utero-oophorectomy (removal of the uterus and ovaries) involves an abdominal incision. Through this incision, both ovaries and both uterine horns are removed to the level of the cervix. With the operation, all female hormonal output from the ovaries is eliminated, as is any influence the uterus might have on whole-body systems. (See The Advantages of Neutering Your Cat on page 116.)

Since this surgery creates an opening into the abdominal cavity, several layers of sutures are used to close the incision. Depending on the technique and suture material used, the outside layer of sutures will usually need to be removed after 7 to 10 days.

THE FEMALE REPRODUCTIVE SYSTEM (NON-NEUTERED CATS)

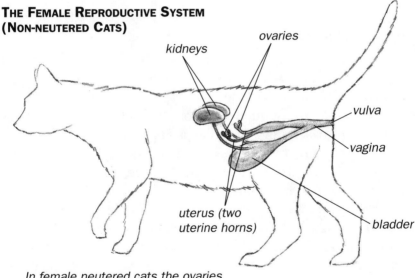

In female neutered cats the ovaries and uterus are removed.

Male neutering, or castration (though this term actually refers to the removal of the reproductive organs), also involves one or two incisions; this time, through the scrotum. After ligating (tying off) the vas deferens and the blood and nerve supplies to the testicles, the surgeon removes the testicles. Sutures may or may not need to be removed, depending on the technique used.

**THE MALE REPRODUCTIVE SYSTEM
(NON-NEUTERED CATS)**

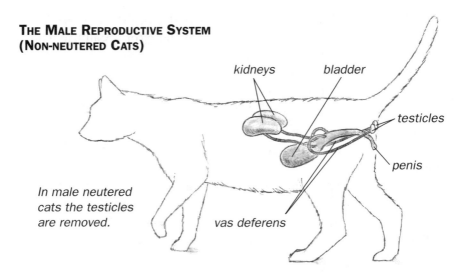

kidneys   bladder

testicles

penis

In male neutered
cats the testicles
are removed.

vas deferens

Why Use Herbs?

To be honest, I don't know many practitioners who agree with my herbs-for-neutered-pets reasoning, and there really isn't much documented scientific evidence to support their use. But I can't help feeling that the sudden and complete loss of primary hormonal organs (ovaries or testes) has a major impact on the entire body, especially the organ systems we know to be responsive to the reproductive hormones (estrogen and testosterone).

When I use herbs, I think I see improvement in some of the problems related to neutering — urinary incontinence and obesity, for instance. Again, I don't have any hard-core documentation, only my clinical observations. Even though I'm out on an unscientific limb, I feel very comfortable recommending herbs for neutered pets because:

- The plants act as organ-system balancers — something I feel the body needs after removing a major source of hormones.
- I think it's the compassionate thing to do; we need to re-supply the hormones we have taken away.
- When used in low doses and as tonics, herbs have very little potential to do harm.
- Although I have only my own positive clinical impressions, I've seen some herbally responsive conditions improve.

- I find that many humans, if they can use herbs to help Pet through the trauma of neutering, feel better about the whole process — which may make it more likely that they will have their next cat neutered.

One Week Pre- and Postsurgery

No matter what the surgery, whenever possible I like to dose the surgery candidate with herbs to help him get through the procedure with a minimum of problems. For about a week pre- and postsurgery I like to give the cat the immune-system balancer echinacea and the antimicrobial Oregon grape root. This is one time when I use a therapeutic dose — a few drops of nonalcoholic tincture 2 or 3 times a day.

Goldenseal can be used in place of Oregon grape root if you can find an organically grown product. Please don't contribute to the precipitous decline of goldenseal in the wild by using unethically harvested plants.

In addition, I recommend a mild tonic, such as nettle leaves, to help activate all systems and provide a ready supply of calcium, vitamin C, and iron.

Finally, I think all animals become anxious when they leave the comforts of their own home, and especially when they are cooped up in a strange cage for a day or two before and after surgery. Valerian root and St.-John's-wort are great antianxiety herbs. Many cats like valerian "in the raw" even better than catnip, so you can simply put some of the root in their dishes and let the cats do the rest. Before the trip to the vet, give your cat a test dose of valerian and catnip to see which one she prefers.

If your cat is responsive to catnip, have the veterinary staff sprinkle a handful of the fresh organic herb on the floor of your cat's recovery-room cage. They can sprinkle the herb 2 to 3 times a day. After your cat returns home, continue the same routine until the sutures are removed,

Valerian

or for 7 to 10 days if suture removal isn't required. After the initial catnip euphoria, cats usually relax and take some extended naptime to sleep it off. Of course, this takes their mind off the pain and misery of the surgery.

After Surgery

After surgery, I supply herbs that might help body systems that are ordinarily influenced by the reproductive hormones. I also try to use herbs that help the whole body. It's especially important to support the following endocrine organs:

- **Adrenals.** Small amounts of reproductive hormones are produced in these glands, and supporting the adrenals, in theory, will help them produce needed amounts of hormones.
- **Thyroid.** My feeling is that the thyroid is almost always secondarily involved in any condition that is hormonally induced (in this case, lack of hormones is the problem).

Herbal Teas for Neutered Pets

I recommend a hormonal tea blend made of equal parts of the selected herbs. The tea should be given once or twice each month throughout your cat's lifetime. The foundation of the teas, whether Pet is male or female, always includes two herbs: licorice root and bladderwrack.

Licorice root works as an adaptogen; it supports all body systems. In addition, it is an herb specific for the adrenals.

Bladderwrack is my other choice because in my experience, hormonally responsive skin conditions in animals go hand-in-hand with an imbalance of thyroid hormones. Bladderwrack is helpful for its thyroid-supportive properties.

> *For the postsurgical male or female cat with anxiety, depression, or inability to sleep, consider using chamomile, wild oat, or valerian root.*

To the licorice root and bladderwrack blend I then select from the herbs discussed next, depending on whether the cat is male or female and on other specific needs he or she may have.

SELECTING HERBS FOR FEMALE CATS

Since we have abruptly removed the cat's source of female hormones, I feel we can serve her needs by resupplying some of these (or their precursors) in a mild and safe herbal form. For example, wild yam contains plant steroids that are precursors in the synthesis of body steroids, such as estrogen and progesterone. Dong quai, Siberian ginseng, and oat are nervines or nervous system tonics that also contain plant steroids that may act as precursors of body steroids.

Wild Yam (Dioscorea villosa)

Wild yam root contains large amounts of plant steroids that are precursors in the synthesis of body steroids, such as estrogen and progesterone. Since their plant steroids have actions similar to those of other steroids in the animal body, yams have long been used for their beneficial effects when treating arthritis.

Dong Quai (Angelica sinensis)

Used as an aid for almost every ailment of the female system, dong quai also helps tone and provide nutrients for the reproductive organs, which makes for an easier hormonal transition. Dong quai is excellent for the circulatory system, is a blood tonic, and is high in minerals, especially iron.

Oat (Avena sativa)

This herb is used for its excellent calming and relaxing (nervine) properties as well as for its plant sterols, which may act as precursors of body steroids, such as estrogen and progesterone. In addition, it is rich in calcium and magnesium.

Nettle (Urtica dioica)

Good as a "booster" for chronic fatigue, nettle is a general tonic for the liver, blood, and nervous system and for glandular imbalances. Nettle is also rich in calcium, iron, and other vitamins and minerals, making this an excellent herb for whole-body nourishment.

Nettle

The Number-One Killer of Pets in the United States

Do you know what single entity in the United States kills more pets than anything else? The answer might surprise you. Euthanasia, or the killing of unwanted pets by lethal injection or electrocution, better known by the euphemism "putting to sleep," ends the lives of more dogs and cats in this country than any disease.

Each year in humane organizations across the United States, millions of dogs and cats (estimates vary from 3 to 10 million or more) are "put to sleep." Many pets are euthanized simply because they are no longer wanted or because they have a behavioral problem; most are not euthanized because they have an incurable disease. Even worse, no one knows how many more animals are euthanized by veterinarians or other individuals.

Since neutering removes the reproductive organs completely, it is the most effective population-control mechanism available. Over time, supposedly better or less-expensive methods have been tried, such as intrauterine devices, injectable chemical sterilization, tubal ligations, and injectable and oral contraceptives. But so far their disadvantages — adverse side effects, difficulty of application, low levels of client interest, and the real inability to greatly reduce the cost of sterilization — have far outweighed their hoped-for advantages.

Occasionally I have a client who asks about tubal ligation (a surgical tie of the oviduct) for the female or vasectomy (ligation of the vas deferens) for the male pet. The problem with these procedures is that they leave the hormone-producers in the body, and we typically neuter Pet because we are interested in more than simple population control.

The tubally ligated female cat will still come into heat, meowing pitifully, wailing, screaming, crying, and caterwauling deep into the night, for days in a row, often joined in a chorus by every tomcat within smelling distance. Then she'll repeat the same-o same-o again and again and again.

Vasectomized male pets, since their testicles are still in there doing their job, retain the urge to mate, roam, fight, and all the other stuff that comes with the testosterone territory.

Chamomile (Anthemis nobilis; Matricaria recutita)

German and Roman chamomile, as well as other related chamomiles, are especially valuable for the neutered female cat who has problems resulting from stress, anxiety, and tension.

Chaste Tree (Vitex agnus-castus)

Chaste tree is typically used in human females to normalize the reproductive tract at all stages of the ovarian cycle, including menopause. It is similarly helpful for cats.

Ginseng (Panax *spp.*)

The ginsengs are among the best all-body tonics and are especially good for stress and fatigue. Although usually considered an herb for males, *Panax* ginseng may be helpful for the timid, cowering female who could use some added yang ("male" characteristics). Siberian ginseng *(Eleutherococcus senticosus)*, not a true ginseng but with similar medicinal uses, is often considered the "female" ginseng. It is good for all systems, especially the circulatory system.

SELECTING HERBS FOR MALE CATS

Much as we can help the neutered female cat, I think that neutered tomcats can benefit from added herbal hormonal precursors. In addition to supporting parts of the body normally helped by male hormones (testosterone), we can offer direct support for the prostate.

Saw Palmetto (Serenoa repens)

Saw palmetto tones and strengthens the male reproductive system. It also increases the tone of the bladder and nourishes the nervous system.

Saw palmetto

Damiania (Turnera diffusa)

This plant acts as a tonic for strengthening the nervous and hormonal systems. It also has antidepressant properties that make it a good herb for treating postneutering anxiety and depression.

Ginseng (Panax *spp.*)

The ginsengs are especially good for stress and fatigue. Most male cats have more than enough yang (male) attributes, so only rarely is *Panax* ginseng indicated. However, Siberian ginseng *(Eleutherococcus sentiocosus)* is an excellent whole-body tonic that can be used for the neutered male cat.

The Advantages of Neutering Your Cat

Without question, the greatest advantage of neutering is that it permanently and completely eliminates your cat's chance to reproduce. In addition, by removing all the reproductive organs and their hormonal impact, we have eliminated (or lessened) many of the secondary aspects of the hormones: heat cycles and all their trials and tribulations in females, and *some* of the roaming and aggression problems inherent in male cats.

Neutering a cat at an early age also greatly decreases his or her chances for developing certain types of tumors. And, of course, with the reproductive organs removed, there is no chance for cancer to develop in those organs.

The Reproductive System (Non-neutered Cats)

I spend so much time and energy trying to get folks to neuter their pets (see the previous chapter) that I sometimes forget that for some families, planned pet parenthood makes perfectly good sense — especially if they have already selected good homes for the future offspring.

Just because your cat hasn't been neutered doesn't mean you shouldn't maintain a holistic health care system, complete with herbal therapies. To help a female or a male cat begin and rear a healthy family:

1. Offer nutritional support — good-quality organic foods with plenty of vitamins and minerals.
2. Create a loving environment in which the cat feels comfortable and relaxed enough to breed (the female cat also needs a comfortable environment in which to give birth and rear her offspring).
3. Enhance the cat's hormonal systems so they can express themselves in a normal fashion; herbal remedies are the natural, effective way to help an animal achieve whole-body hormonal balance.

For cats with reproductive problems or other specific male or female diseases, I use a combination of chiropractic and acupuncture. The results I achieve with these two methods are often amazing. In addition, many of the gender-related problems respond favorably to homeopathic remedies. To support these therapies, I add herbal remedies and pay attention to the cat's diet and stress levels.

HERBAL ENHANCERS FOR FEMALE CATS

I like to use ½ cup of mild tea for the mother-to-be, poured over her food several times a week throughout the breeding years. Ideally the tea should contain hormonal or specific sex-organ tonics (such as uterine and ovarian tonics), enhance liver function (the liver is the site of production and metabolism of many of the body's hormones), and provide a healthy abundance of vitamins and minerals. For female cats, choose two or more herbs from the following list.

Dong Quai (Angelica sinensis)

This herb is excellent for use over an extended period of time to strengthen and balance the uterus. Dong quai has no specific hormonal action; it helps regulate and balance hormonal production via its liver-cleansing and blood-nourishing activities. The plant is also a mild nervine, helping calm and relax nervous Nellies.

Wild Yam (Dioscorea villosa)

Wild yam contains steroidal precursors that have been used for years to provide the building blocks for a variety of steroidal drugs, including birth control pills and cortisone. Long before its use in drug manufacturing, wild yam was used by herbalists to normalize hormone production; it helps regulate the ratio of progesterone to estrogen in the body. Wild yam is also a liver tonic, and it has anti-inflammatory activity.

Chaste Tree (Vitex agnus-castus)

Depending on which of the various folklore claims you read, you might think that this herb's major activity is suppressing libido.

But according to the French herbalist Cazin, the herb is sexually stimulating. The truth is, however, that chaste tree is neither stimulating nor suppressing. It is a normalizing herb that works through the pituitary gland to regulate female (and male) sex hormones. It is excellent for restoring and regulating the female's estrogen-progesterone balance. It has no known side effects, so it can be used for prolonged periods.

Chaste tree

Black Cohosh (Cimicifuga recemosa)

Although they are unrelated, black and blue cohosh are often used in combination for their synergistic effects. Black cohosh has an estrogen-like effect and is used to balance and regulate female hormones. During labor it may be used to aid uterine activity while relieving nervousness.

Blue Cohosh (Caulophyllum thalictroides)

Also known as squaw root or papoose root, this herb was used by Native American women during the later stages of pregnancy to ensure easy labor and delivery. Today's herbalists consider blue cohosh one of the best uterine stimulants available. It is also a potent antispasmodic that can be used to relieve coughs, asthma, and arthritic pain. Since it may cause premature uterine contractions, it should not be used in the early stages of pregnancy.

Nettle (Urtica dioica)

Nettle is valuable as both a food and a medicine. It is considered by many to be a gourmet green and is lightly steamed and used as a salad or cooked and eaten like spinach. Nettle is high in vitamins and minerals, especially calcium, iron, and vitamin C. An herbal medicine that strengthens and supports the entire body, nettle has a strong reputation as a pregnancy tonic, an antihemorrhagic during childbirth, and a therapy for a variety of female problems. It can also be used to enrich and increase milk flow and to restore and rebuild the mother's energy after childbirth.

Raspberry (Rubus idaeus)

Known to herbalists as the herb supreme for pregnant women, raspberry leaf has a long tradition of use during pregnancy to strengthen and tone uterine tissue. It's also used to assist in contractions and prevent hemorrhaging during labor. Raspberry leaves contain high amounts of vitamins and minerals, especially calcium and iron. Raspberry is safe to use during all stages of pregnancy.

> ### LIVER HELPERS
>
> To enhance the production and metabolism of hormones, whether your cat is male or female, include one or more of the liver-helper herbs: milk thistle, dandelion, turmeric. For more information on liver herbs, see chapter 14.

Milk-Flow Enhancers

If your new mother cat needs a little help in getting the milk flowing, try one of these herbs:

Fenugreek

- **Fennel** *(Foeniculum vulgare)*. The seeds of this plant are probably the best herb for increasing milk flow. Fennel is also excellent for colic and flatulence and has been used to treat coughs and bronchitis.
- **Fenugreek** *(Trigonella foenum-graecum)*. Another good herb for stimulating milk flow, fenugreek seed is also used to ease sore throats and bronchitis. Externally, it will treat sores and wounds.
- **Blessed thistle** *(Cnicus benedictus)*. The leaves of this plant enhance milk flow. However, the herb is also a digestion-enhancing bitter. Most cats hate the taste of bitters, so I usually use fennel and fenugreek.

Herbs to Avoid during Pregnancy

Several herbs stimulate the uterus, and the resultant uterine contractions (which can be helpful during other times of the female cycle) can cause abortion. Avoid giving your pregnant cat the following herbs.

- Arborvitae (*Thuja* spp.)
- Barberry (*Berberis* spp.)
- Goldenseal *(Hydrastis canadensis)*
- Juniper *(Juniperus communis)*
- Male fern *(Dryopteris crassirhizoma)*
- Pennyroyal *(Mentha pulegium)*
- Poke root *(Phytolacca americana)*
- Rue *(Ruta graveolens)*
- Sage *(Salvia officinalis)*
- Southernwood *(Artemisia abrotanum)*
- Tansy *(Tanacetum vulgare)*
- Wormwood *(Artemisia absinthium)*

Mammary Cancers

Mammary cancers are almost always nasty in cats. When there is a palpable growth in the mammary region, I recommend immediate surgical removal of the mass along with a biopsy to help determine the cat's prognosis. After tumor removal, herbs may be helpful in preventing recurrence. I have tried some of the herbs with supposed anticancer activity, so far with varying amounts of success. Herbs to consider include echinacea, goldenseal, chaparral, noni juice, and aloe vera. See chapter 8 for more information on herbs for cancer.

HERBAL ENHANCERS FOR MALE CATS

As with intact female cats, non-neutered male cats benefit from ½ cup of mild tea poured over the food several times a week throughout the breeding years. This tea should include hormonal or specific sex-organ tonics (such as testicular tonics). Enhancing liver function and providing vitamins and minerals are goals of male herbal therapy, as well. Here are some herbal helpers for the male cat.

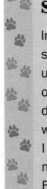

SPRAYING

Intact male cats almost always spray; it's a natural habit they use to mark their territory with odiferous urine. Sorry, but I don't know of any herbs that will prevent this habit, nor do I know of any plants that will make the urine smell better. For the spraying tomcat, castration is the only effective treatment I know.

Damiana (Turnera diffusa)

Damiana has an ancient reputation as an aphrodisiac. Perhaps this is true; more important, the herb acts as a nervous tonic, an antidepressant, a urinary antiseptic, and a laxative. Also, it contains alkaloids that have testosterone-like action, apparently strengthening the male reproductive system.

Saw Palmetto (Serenoa repens)

Saw palmetto berries tone and strengthen the male reproductive system. They can be used safely when a boost of male sexual hormones is needed.

Male Reproductive Problems

It's my observation that most male cats don't need much help in boosting their libido or their reproductive capacities. However, if you have the rare cat with breeding reluctance I recommend improving the diet, adding vitamin E and selenium, and using tonic herbs in combination with mild herbal nervines to alleviate stress and anxiety factors. The initial nervine herbs I consider are oat, hop, and chamomile. In addition, try liver or general tonics, such as nettle, dandelion root, milk thistle, Siberian ginseng, and licorice root.

The Respiratory System

The respiratory system is the method by which your cat communicates with the flow of nature. With each contraction of his muscular diaphragm, your cat draws in volumes of raw air — air with its nourishing oxygen, its wonderful aromas, the essences of local herbs . . . and all the area's pollutants.

The air first passes through an intricate labyrinth of mucus-lined tissues in your cat's nose, and then travels down a long tube (trachea), into smaller tubes (bronchi), and finally into the microscopic chambers (alveoli) of the lung. Within the alveoli the air is processed; oxygen is then picked up by the red blood cells coursing through the many blood vessels that line the alveoli, and carbon dioxide is passed outward to be eliminated during expiration.

Along the way, the inspired air passes through a maze of structures, many of which are coated with mucus and lined with tiny hairs that constantly beat outward. These structures filter out the "bad-guy" stuff. At each step along its journey, the inhaled air also experiences a complex system of immune-system checks and

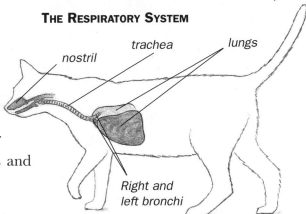

THE RESPIRATORY SYSTEM

nostril

trachea

lungs

Right and left bronchi

balances. The natural way for a cat to expel foreign material is to sneeze and cough, so a certain amount of these activities is a natural way to keep the system clean and healthy.

RESPIRATORY DISEASE

For a healthy cat there's nothing better than a breath of fresh air; for a cat with respiratory system disease, breathing may be almost impossible. Respiratory diseases can occur all along the system — from the nose (rhinitis) to the trachea (tracheitis) through the bronchi (bronchitis) and into the lungs (pneumonia).

Causes

Causes of respiratory disease are many: bacterial, viral, and fungal infections; parasites; cancers; and infiltration of pollutants. Cigarette tars are a big culprit here; if you smoke, quit — if not for your own health, then for your cat's. Upper respiratory disease is very common in cats, especially kittens. A whole host of viruses can cause infection of the nose and sinuses (sneezing and nasal discharge are frequently symptoms), and secondary bacterial infections are common companions. Asthma is also a common finding.

What Are the Symptoms?

Symptoms of disease in the respiratory system include:

- Shortness of breath
- Difficulty breathing
- Excess coughing and sneezing
- Discharge from the nose

A stethoscope will help your vet hear abnormalities, such as rough or raspy breathing patterns, fluid, or dead areas that indicate a total lack of air movement. As with any other health problem, professional diagnosis is critical.

Cats and Respiratory Disease

Cats with upper respiratory infections are easy to diagnose: They have runny eyes, sneezing, discharge from the nose. Since these infections are most often viral, herbs are my first treatment of choice.

When a cat comes to me with a chronic respiratory problem, I first consider asthma. Second, I check for the possibility of heart disease. Then I consider chronic viral infection that has lingered from a past upper respiratory infection. Next, I ask whether there are smokers in the house. Secondary smoke is as harmful to your cat as it is to you. Finally, I address the possibility of cancer. Primary lung tumors can occur, but more common are neoplasias (tumors) that have their origins in another organ and have subsequently spread to the lungs. X rays are indicated to rule out cancer.

If none of these problems is present, I almost always find that a chronic cough is due to a lack of balance in the cat's immune system. In those cases, I take a standard holistic approach to treatment.

THE HOLISTIC APPROACH

A good holistic protocol for treating respiratory disease starts with getting rid of irritants. Sometimes it's also necessary to use cough suppressants. Once irritated tissues are soothed, we can reestablish a normal air flow through the lungs with good oxygen/carbon dioxide exchange into the bloodstream. Finally, I use herbs to balance the immune system, which helps stave off permanent damage from the disease.

Herbal medicines have been a healthy addition to the arsenal I use to combat respiratory problems. I have found that acupuncture is often helpful for difficult cases, especially asthma, and I always evaluate animals chiropractically to be sure there is not a spinal or rib problem that may be hindering respiration. But many of the respiratory cases I see, both chronic and acute, respond very well to herbs alone.

Step 1: Eliminate Irritants

First, examine the general lifestyle of the people and animals in your household. Does anyone smoke? Do you use any chemicals for outdoor or indoor chores, or special powders and sprays for gardening or cleaning? Exposure to any of these irritants can prompt respiratory problems in cats. Rarely, foreign bodies that have found their way into the different parts of the respiratory tract can be culprits.

In addition to eliminating environmental irritants, antimicrobial herbs can be used to enhance the immune system's response. A combination of echinacea and goldenseal (or Oregon grape root) in a tea, tincture, or capsule/tablet is hard to beat. These herbs have mild antimicrobial activity, and echinacea is an immune-system stimulant. You can even add thyme for additional antimicrobial action.

Goldenseal

Step 2: Suppress Excess Coughing

Licorice root *(Glycyrrhiza glabra)* in tincture or tea form works well as a suppressant for coughs that seem to be located in the throat, larynx, or upper respiratory areas. Licorice root is also helpful for strengthening the respiratory system.

Mullein *(Verbascum thapsus)* is good for deeper, dry coughs. This plant suppresses coughs and acts as a lung tonic. Use it as a tea, or put some fresh mullein in a cool mist humidifier and let it run for several hours in the room where your cat normally sleeps (overnight is perfect). Smudging, or lighting a bundle of dried herb leaves and then letting them burn so that the smoke permeates the room, is a traditional way to treat lung problems. Mullein can be used in this way; in fact, one of its common names, bullock's lungwort, comes from the traditional practice of smudging the herb to treat herds of cows.

Thyme *(Thymus vulgaris)*, in addition to having mild antimicrobial activity, helps relieve the spasms that are characteristic of coughs.

Osha root *(Ligusticum porteri)* is a traditional herb used by Native Americans in the southwestern United States to treat colds, flu, and other upper respiratory infections.

Coltsfoot *(Tussilago farfara)* has a soothing effect. It also acts as an expectorant, helping to move mucus out of the system. An anti-inflammatory, coltsfoot is a good herb to consider for either acute or chronic conditions.

Step 3: Soothe Irritated Tissues

Marsh mallow root and slippery elm bark are both soothing to all mucous

> *Cats with decreased adrenal function are more susceptible to developing chronic coughs. Licorice root is specific for the adrenal glands.*

membranes, and they work well to ease a dry cough. (Use coltsfoot, thyme, osha, or licorice for a wet cough.) Turmeric has natural anti-inflammatory activity, and it will strengthen immune function. As a natural diuretic, nettle will help dry out congested sinuses, and its hearty content of vitamins and minerals will speed healing.

Step 4: Reestablish Normal Air Flow

In order to reestablish normal air flow through the lungs with good oxygen/carbon dioxide exchange into the bloodstream, try these helpful herbs:

Ginkgo *(Ginkgo biloba)* has antiallergy and antiasthmatic activity. It also relieves constriction of the bronchi.

Ephedra *(Ephedra sinica)* is a bronchodilator that is useful for asthma, bronchitis, and allergic problems related to the respiratory system. This herb is also known as ma huang in Chinese medicine. It attained recent notoriety when the pharmaceutical version was implicated in several human deaths. But the problem was that the drug was contaminated with excess ephedra and perhaps other drugs. This is simply one more case that supports my reluctance to use Chinese herbs — it is almost impossible to rely on their purity or quality.

Step 5: Balance the Immune System

Echinacea *(Echinacea* spp.) is my favorite immune-balancing herb. During acute bouts of coughing, I suggest therapeutic (i.e., high) doses of the herb, given orally as a tincture or capsule/tablet. For chronic coughs, I recommend echinacea, again in tincture or capsule or tablet form, used in an on/off schedule — 3 weeks on, 1 week off, then repeat as indicated.

Astragalus *(Astragalus membranaceus)* enhances the immune system and helps strengthen the lungs. Astragalus also stimulates the regeneration of bronchial cells.

Licorice root *(Glycyrrhiza glabra)*, along with supplemental pantothenic acid, enhances the functioning of the adrenals, the master glands of the immune system. Pantothenic acid is readily available as the supplement calcium pantothenate and is also available from many food sources, including brewer's yeast, liver, peanuts, mushrooms, soybeans, peas, oatmeal, and sunflower seeds.

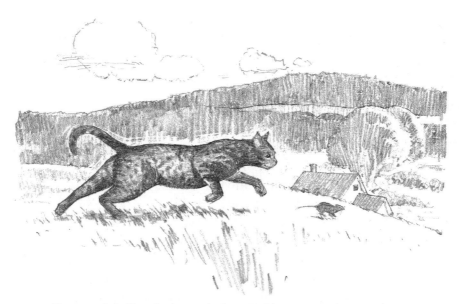

If your cat suffers from respiratory problems, exercise may be difficult for him. Try herbal remedies to restore easy breathing.

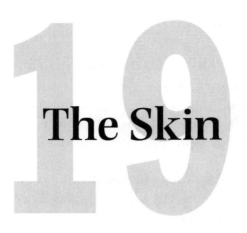

The Skin

I see three types of skin conditions routinely in my practice: the generally easy-to-fix superficial scrapes, cuts, and abrasions; skin problems related to external parasites, such as fleas and mange mites; and chronic skin conditions from "who knows where."

The superficial nicks and cuts respond extremely well to herbal medications; so well, in fact, that I routinely recommend them in lieu of anything else. Skin problems related to parasites often respond well to herbal remedies — once we have eliminated the parasite with a chemical treatment. I do not find herbs especially effective against any type of parasite, external or internal.

Chronic skin conditions from "who knows where" sometimes respond to herbs, but these problems are my biggest bugaboo. They are well at the top of my list of daily frustrating cases, no matter which "magic medicine" I try. However, some of these tough cases actually do respond well to herbs, so I continue to approach each individual case with hope and prayer — and a healthy arsenal of herbs, acupuncture, homeopathy, nutritional supplements, chiropractic adjustments, and whatever else I can think of.

HERBS FOR SUPERFICIAL SKIN LESIONS

Let's start with the easy-to-fix superficial skin lesions. There's a whole potpourri of herbs that can be used on minor cuts, scrapes, and open wounds. Commercial products often incorporate one or more of these herbs into salves, ointments, unguents, oils, sprays, and so forth.

Liberally apply the salves, ointments, or oils to wounds that look like they could use some softening. Use natural products, and stay away from any product that contains an ingredient you can't pronounce. I highly recommend homemade products.

On a skin area that is red, inflamed, and oozing, use a liquid-based product that will help dry the area. I like to brew a tea of one or more healing herbs and spritz it directly onto the affected area several times a day. The tea can be kept in the refrigerator for a few days; then brew up another batch.

ACNE: A SPECIAL CAT SKIN PROBLEM

Although I've seen this condition on dogs a time or two, it more often appears on cats. Acne typically appears on the cat's lower chin, and it may spread to other parts of the face. The condition usually consists of small, raised, pustulelike areas that feel hard to the touch. We don't really know what causes the lesions — it's one of those from "who knows where" skin problems — but Western medicine tries to fix them with an arsenal of chemicals, including hormones and antibiotics.

I've had good results getting rid of acne with herbs; I simply choose from my "who knows where" skin herbs. Typically, I use echinacea, Oregon grape root, licorice root, burdock root, red clover, sarsaparilla, and yellow dock. I also recommend topical skin herbs; choose from the list on pages 131–132.

Also, I should mention that I've seen several cases of acne clear up when we replace the cat's plastic water and food dishes with glass or porcelain. Is it an allergy-related disease? Good possibility.

Calendula (Calendula officinalis)

Calendula contains the pain-relieving compound salicylic acid (also found in aspirin) and has anti-inflammatory, antiviral, antibacterial, and antifungal activity. Calendula also speeds wound healing by enhancing epithelial tissue growth. In addition to applying it externally, we can use calendula internally for its anti-microbial effects as well as its ability to enhance liver function.

Aloe (Aloe vera)

Use the fresh juice of aloe for wounds and especially for burns and sunburn. Keep a plant in the house at all times so that you have a constant supply of fresh leaves. Then, when you need aloe's healing powers, simply break off a leaf and squeeze its juice onto the wound. Don't use it internally, since too much can act as a cathartic (laxative).

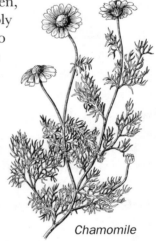

Chamomile (Anthemis nobilis; Matricaria recutita)

While its internal calming effects are well known, chamomile also seems to calm a pet's anxiety when it is used topically. Chamomile speeds wound healing and is especially good for inflamed lesions.

Chamomile

Other Herbs

Lavender aids healing, relieves anxiety, and eases aches and pains.

Mullein speeds healing and is soothing to inflamed areas.

Plantain has gentle healing qualities. The leaf, used as a poultice, will act as a "drawing agent," helping to remove foreign bodies buried deep in wounds.

St.-John's-wort not only eases pain but also helps speed the healing of wounds, bruises, and mild burns.

Yarrow is an excellent healing herb. It will also stop the bleeding from oozing wounds.

WHAT TO DO ABOUT LICKING

Most cats will try to lick off any medication applied topically. Since the herbs mentioned here can be used internally, consuming them won't hurt your cat at all. (On commercial products, remember to read the label ingredients, and be sure the herbs are in an all-natural base.) But by removing the medication, the effectiveness is decreased. A pinch of cayenne added to each application of the ointment may help prevent licking, and cayenne is currently being studied for its anti-pain and wound-healing capabilities.

About Abscesses

Cats, especially tomcats, are territorial, and they'll fight off any prowlers who happen to be on their turf. Usually these are merely spit-and-huff tiffs, but some confrontations end up as full-fledged brawls. Cat abscesses, or fluid-filled lumps under the skin, are a common result.

You'll know your cat has an abscess when he becomes lethargic. He may not eat, and he will often act as if it's a big problem just to walk about. You may be able to find the abscess, and you may even be able to feel a scab over the entry point where the victorious cat's teeth or claws initially penetrated.

The lump is actually filled with pus — nasty-smelling, evil-looking stuff often produced in unimaginable quantities. Fortunately, the abscess usually looks (and smells) much worse than it is in terms of how it affects your cat. In fact, if left alone, most abscesses rupture and drain, then heal on their own. But most of us want to help our cats get over pain and misery as quickly as possible.

I almost always open the abscess (usually under general anesthesia), drain it of its exudate, flush it with hydrogen peroxide or antibiotics, and then leave a fairly large opening so that the pus can continue to drain. I also give the cat a healthy internal dose of antibiotics. But if you prefer using herbal medicines, I've had good results with those, too.

For an herbal abscess treatment, I first make a small incision to open the skin for drainage. I then have the client pack the incision with a poultice of plantain several times a day for several days.

Plantain helps draw out the pus, allowing a better area for healing. This is important because other herbs, such as calendula, will cause the drainage site to rapidly heal over, creating another abscess. After each plantain treatment we'll flush the abscess site with hydrogen peroxide, then follow up by flushing with warm tea made from one or more of the topical skin herbs (calendula, yarrow, mullein, or chamomile). We also give the cat a 1- to 2-week regimen of internal antibiotic herbs; I prefer echinacea combined with yarrow, Oregon grape root, calendula, thyme, and/or chamomile.

HERBS FOR PARASITE-RELATED PROBLEMS

The most common offender here is the lowly flea. Although cats are not nearly as suscept-ible to fleas as their canine counterparts, fleas can still be a problem. The key, of course, is to eliminate the flea. I haven't found an herb that is effective for this, so the main thrust of my herbal approach is to enhance the cat's immune system while helping the gen-eral health of the skin.

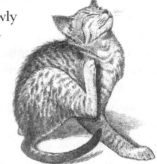

The itching caused by fleas will make your cat scratch quite frequently.

Echinacea (Echinacea *spp.*)

The primary herb to use for immune enhancement is echinacea. I like to dose echinacea in an on/off way: use daily for 3 weeks, then take 1 week off; repeat as needed. Or use it for 5 days, then take 2 days off; repeat as needed.

Diet

If you look at a typical family of animals, it always seems that there's one poor critter that has all the fleas and almost all the skin (and other health) problems. I'm not sure what this means, but I *think* it means that the poor soul has a deficient immune system. Improved diet and immune-balancing herbs are often helpful.

I've had many clients swear that their cat was rid of all its fleas after they added brewer's yeast to the diet. On the other hand, researchers who study fleas and keep colonies of them alive so they can do the studies tell me that their preferred flea food is brewer's yeast. Go figure. In any event, an addition of brewer's yeast isn't going to hurt, and it may provide just the nutrient boost your cat needs.

Herbs for Chronic and Iatrogenic Skin Conditions

Skin conditions can come from so many different directions: bacterial or fungal infections; nutritional, hormonal, or immune system imbalances; spinal nerve impingement; hereditary causes; and many other things that come under the heading of chronic, idiopathic ("we have absolutely no idea what causes this") conditions.

Another type of skin condition is referred to as iatrogenic. Iatrogenic means "doctor caused," but, in truth, these diseases are usually caused by doctors using the medicines they learned to use in their Western training. In other words, iatrogenic diseases are caused by the toxic effects of drugs.

With this in mind, it should be clear that a good diagnosis is imperative before you'll know which way to proceed with the herbs. Find a veterinarian who goes beyond the obligatory, quick-fix cortisone-shot-and-a-flea-collar method. Find one who gives your cat a thorough dermatologic workup, including skin scrapings and cultures, blood tests, and biopsies when necessary. After the vet check, you can use herbs that support other therapeutic methods. Some herbs will help create and maintain healthy skin and haircoats while we await the rare miracle.

With the veritable plethora of causes that can contribute to skin ailments, there are as many herbs that may apply to your cat's particular skin condition. Here are some of my favorite skin herbs.

Licorice (Glycyrrhiza glabra)

This herb finds its way into most of my herbal formulations because of its adaptogenic qualities; it is beneficial to all organ systems. And since most cats like its taste, licorice is a good choice for camouflaging the bitter taste of other herbs. In addition, licorice root specifically aids the adrenal glands, which produce natural cortisone. Therefore, I use it for any condition where I might once have used cortisone — and especially for skin conditions.

Burdock (Arctium lappa)

Burdock acts as a "blood cleanser," promoting excretion of wastes in the urine and sweat. It is a valuable remedy for skin conditions, especially those in which the skin is dry and scaly. Since some herbalists report a synergy between red clover *(Trifolium pratense)* and burdock, I usually combine the two in approximately equal portions.

Sarsaparilla (Smilax *spp.*)

Sarsaparilla is especially good for diffuse systemic problems, such as chronic skin conditions. In addition, sarsaparilla is indicated for other chronic systemic conditions, such as arthritis, and it has antibacterial actions for skin (or other) conditions caused by bacteria.

Yellow Dock (Rumex crispus)

Used extensively in the treatment of chronic skin problems, yellow dock, like burdock root, also benefits the liver. Yellow dock aids in the elimination of toxins that may be responsible for skin conditions.

Sarsaparilla

Other Herbs

Burdock root, yellow dock, and sarsaparilla (with red clover added for good measure) are my triumvirate of primary skin herbs. But since the skin is affected by so many other organ systems, we also need to consider them in our holistic approach to skin problems.

For example, many of the skin cases I see occur in the "couch potato" cat. Lack of exercise makes for poor circulation and stagnant blood, both of which can cause unhealthy skin. Besides recommending daily exercise, I try **nettle,** which is a blood stimulator and has been used in people as a springtime tonic to clear up chronic skin ailments.

The liver is also a critical organ for clearing internal toxins that may be causing skin irritation. And so I might add a liver tonic, such as **dandelion** or **chicory,** to my herbal remedy. Or if symptoms indicate that the liver may be a primary organ of concern, I add **milk thistle.**

It's my belief that all problems of the skin either initially or ultimately have an adverse effect on the immune system; herbs that rebalance immunity are always beneficial. **Echinacea** is my mainstay for helping the immune system, and it appears in nearly all of my skin remedies. If the skin condition is complicated by a bacterial infection, I add some of the antibacterial herbs, such as calendula or Oregon grape root.

Finally, think about your cat and how difficult it must be for him to deal with the infernal itching and scratching. Some of the cats I see have been literally driven crazy by the constant irritation. I think we need to do all we can to ease Pet's mental duress. Some mind herbs that I find helpful include:

- St.-John's-wort, for its ability to alleviate irritability and anxiety, and for its healing and anti-pain characteristics
- Oat, for the cat who seems to need just a little calming
- Valerian, if your cat seems almost paranoid, worrying about his itching
- Chamomile, if he can't get any sleep

CASE STUDY

I remember Charlotte, a seven-year-old long-haired domestic (mixed-breed) female cat. We were treating Charlotte for her primary problem, inflammatory bowel disease, and we considered her skin condition secondary. For several years Charlotte had suffered with a chronic skin condition that periodically had nearly driven her crazy with intense itching over the shoulders, along the belly and into the flank, and across the neck. She would dig at herself until her claws made deep scratches across the length of her neck, and the areas she could lick were bald and raw.

We put Charlotte on my protocol for inflammatory bowel disease (see chapter 12) and within two weeks her chronic diarrhea had stopped — and so had her itching. On her first follow-up visit she no longer had raw areas on her back, neck, and belly, and her hair was already starting to grow back.

Indicator Lawns

Many years ago I learned about lawn care and its impact on skin health after I'd been unsuccessfully treating a client's dogs for a recurrent allergic skin condition that periodically cropped up on their belly, legs, and paws. One of her dogs also had a small infected area between its toes that appeared to be due to a splinter — the perfect candidate for a drawing poultice of plantain leaf. The client also had a cat with early liver and kidney problems that I thought could benefit from dandelion root tea.

Thinking that this would be a great time to demonstrate the power of backyard weeds, we walked out her back door, where I planned to show her how to harvest and use nature's medicines. After a lengthy search of her well-manicured lawn, and after finding not one weed, we checked the front yard. Again, nary a weed.

Then the light struck the dim abyss of my brain. "You have a lawn care service, don't you?" I asked.

"Why, yes, we most certainly do," she answered, rather haughtily.

No weeds — none of nature's beautiful, healing plants. The culprit: heavy doses of pesticides and herbicides, toxic chemicals that may lead to allergic reactions — exactly like the skin problems this lady's dogs had been dealing with for years. Not surprisingly, the periodic nature of the skin irritations corresponded with the visits from the lawn service. When we got rid of the lawn service, the skin allergies disappeared . . . and my herb and acupuncture treatments looked like true miracles.

Ever since that eye-opener, I've made it a point to check my clients' lawns for weedy "indicator" plants. They can tell me much about a pet's state of health.

The Thyroid

Don't be surprised if your veterinarian tells you that your cat's thyroid isn't functioning properly. Every year I see more and more cases of thyroid imbalance in animals. In cats the most common problem is hyperthyroidism (overproduction of thyroxin), usually caused by a tumor of the thyroid. The tumor is usually a benign tumor called an adenoma.

ABOUT THE THYROID

For such a wee gland, the thyroid has a mighty big effect on your cat's entire body. Thyroxin, the hormone produced by a bean-sized chunk of thyroidal glandular tissue located along your cat's neck, energizes cellular reactions and increases oxygen consumption in the trillions of cells located in all parts of the body. So an imbalance of thyroid hormone produces myriad symptoms throughout the body.

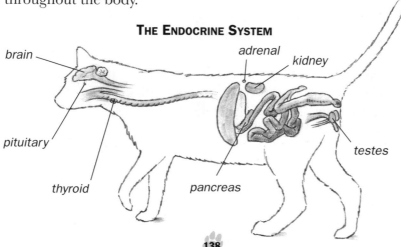

THE ENDOCRINE SYSTEM

brain

adrenal

kidney

pituitary

testes

thyroid

pancreas

Possible Causes of Hyperthryoidism

Why are we seeing such an increase of thyroid disease in cats, dogs, and other animals? Unfortunately, there is no simple, one-cause answer, especially when we are talking about such a complex disease as cancer. Evidently, the thyroid is a target organ for many outside influences, and our modern world may have much to do with our cats' thyroid problems.

For example, immune-mediated causes are often implicated in cancers. Stress, which produces internal cortisol, decreases the amount of thyroxin available and may ultimately cause abnormal cell growth. Any kind of external cortisone therapy will, of course, also have the same effect. Lack of exercise decreases thyroxin production, and how many cats do we know today that get enough exercise?

> *Whether a cat has hyper- or hypothyroidism, my approach is to always try holistic treatments first before going to the Western medicine extremes of surgery or hormone replacement therapy.*

Many nutritional factors may affect thyroid function as well. For example, the thyroid requires iodine to function, but an excess can be toxic. Selenium is also a required mineral; but once again, too much can be toxic. Tyrosine is the necessary amino acid building block for thyroxine, and therefore its sources must be available in the diet. (See the box Foods for Thyroid Disease on page 141.)

Holistic practitioners feel that exposure to toxic chemicals, pesticides, herbicides, preservatives in foods, heavy metals (especially mercury), and possibly even excess vaccines (see the Consumer Alert box on page 145) may compromise the thyroid, leading to the autoimmune reactions that cause disease. And since we often see a high incidence of thyroid disease occurring along a whole blood-line of pets, we can conclude that it can also be genetically linked.

Symptoms of Hyperthyroidism

Although hyperthyroidism can occur in all animals, it is most common in middle-aged to old cats. The most common cause is a thyroid adenoma (cancer). The symptoms that can occur with an increased amount of thyroxin, as you'd expect, reflect a metabolism that has run amok:

- Increased appetite
- Weight loss
- Hyperexcitability
- Increased thirst
- Increased urination

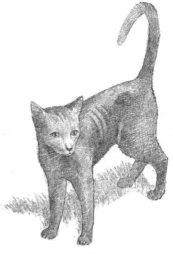

Many animals also have gastro-intestinal upsets, such as vomiting and diarrhea, and some experience an increased heart rate that, if extreme, can be life threatening. The thyroid may become enlarged enough for you to palpate it in the neck.

Many of the cats I've seen with hyperthyroidism have the above symptoms in excess. They will eat as if they haven't had a meal in the past four

Hyperthyroid cats may lose weight quickly and exhibit hyperexcitability.

weeks, and as soon as they're done, they'll eat again. And they still lose weight. It seems that no matter how ravenous their appetite, they gradually deteriorate to skin and bones. Your cat may also be a nervous wreck, pacing the floor at all hours, whining and wailing. Many have on-and-off bouts of diarrhea, sometimes severe. Increased heart rate and increased intensity are both common symptoms in cats with hyperthyroidism.

Treating Thyroid Imbalance

Conventional therapy for hyperthyroidism consists of some method of destroying the thyroid — chemical treatment (with methimazole, for example), surgical removal, or "nuke" treatment (chemotherapy, such as radioactive iodine). In addition, for the many hyperthyroid cats that have increased heart rates, a drug (such as propranolol or Inderal) is administered to slow the heart.

But once you've destroyed or surgically removed the thyroid, it is no longer there (duh!). Your only hope at this stage is to try to restore the thyroid's long list of normal functions with synthetic doses of hormones. In a practical sense, this is not always possible. So I discourage this approach unless it is absolutely necessary.

As a holistic veterinarian, I think we are meowing up the wrong tree when we say that cancer causes hyperthyroidism in cats. I think that some abnormal stimulus (or combination of abnormal stimuli)

Foods for Thyroid Disease

When I'm treating mild to moderate cases of hyperthyroidism, raw cruciferous vegetables are helpful because they contain a natural thyroid blocker. Examples of this type of plant include broccoli, cauliflower, cabbage, kale, collards, Brussels sprouts, and mustard greens. While most cats don't exactly relish these veggies, I've found that many of them will tolerate small amounts ground into gruel in a food blender and then mixed into their food.

For the hypothyroid cat, you'll need to add small amounts of iodine, zinc, copper, and tyrosine to the diet to stimulate and support the thyroid.

- **Iodine** sources include the seaweeds listed on pages 144–145 and sea salt. Iodized salt is also a source, but not the best because it usually contains aluminum. Cod-liver oil also contains traces of iodine. Many areas of our seas have been contaminated with heavy metals, so knowing the source of your sea herbs and salts is important.
- **Zinc** sources include beef, oatmeal, chicken, seafood (especially oysters and tuna), liver, beans, bran, spinach, seeds, and nuts.
- **Copper** can be found in liver and other organ meats, eggs, yeast, legumes, nuts, and raisins.
- **Tyrosine** (from phenylalanine, another amino acid) is found in soy products, beef, chicken, and fish.

causes an imbalance in Kitty's thyroid, which then leads to an abnormal growth of thyroidal cells — better known as cancer. I am totally convinced that it is one or a combination of outside factors (mentioned previously) that is causing the tremendous increase in the cases of thyroid imbalance we practitioners are seeing today. And so I treat all cases of thyroid imbalance — both hyper- and hypothyroidism — by trying to bring the gland back into balance.

Holistic treatment of a thyroid imbalance includes nutritional adjustments, proper exercise, removal of possible causes of toxicity (including drugs), and minimization of stress. In the case of hypothyroidism, appropriate thyroid supplementation is necessary. In the case of hyperthyroidism, though, foods are used to suppress thyroid activity. (See the box Foods for Thyroid Disease on page 141.)

I've had the most success treating both hypo- or hyperthyroidism when I've added either constitutional homeopathy or acupuncture to my overall treatment regimen, which always includes herbs to supplement the holistic therapy.

DIAGNOSTIC TESTS FOR THYROID DISEASE

The common form of thyroid disease in cats, hyperthyroidism, is relatively easy to diagnose; there's a simple blood test that can be used to correlate symptoms with excess thyroxin (T-4) production.

Diagnosing hypothyroidism is a little more difficult. Without getting into a bunch of medical mumbo-jumbo, let's just say that to accurately diagnose hypothyroidism you'll need at least two tests — the T-4 and the thyroid-stimulating test. Have the results of both of these analyzed by a holistic veterinarian *before* you resort to Western medicine's confrontational treatments.

I've had reasonable success treating both hyper- and hypothyroidism with alternative medicines only. But I have noticed that in some of the animals I am treating, even though their symptoms have disappeared — that is, by all external appearances they have returned to a normally functioning critter — T-4 levels may remain abnormal for several months. I caution folks that we may need to wait at least several months before the blood tests return to normal.

HERBS FOR HYPERTHYROIDISM

Herbs are the perfect adjunct to a holistic treatment of hyperthyroidism. Remember that the last thing we want to do is to totally remove the thyroid and all its beneficial actions. We want to slow it back down to a more normal level of function. In addition, since hyperthyroid cats typically have increased heart rates, we need to add herbs to slow the heart rate and to help balance overall cardiac function.

Patience is a key word when treating hyperthyroidism holistically. It may take a few months to get the thyroid back into balance. (I don't like to see the heart race along for months at a time, so if the cardiac herbs don't work to slow the heart rate in 3 to 4 weeks, I usually suggest we go to Western cardiac drugs. And don't expect blood values to change right away after herbal treatments begin. I'm not sure why this is, but I've had several cases of hyperthyroidism that have kept high levels of thyroxin for months or years, even though *all* the symptoms of hyperthyroidism have long since disappeared.

Bugleweed (Lycopus virginicus, L. europaeus)

Bugleweed is a specific herb to moderate the overactive thyroid. In addition, it is a heart tonic, used to strengthen that organ and reduce its rate. Bugleweed is also a valuable sedative, helping to relax the cat who is hyperactive from excess thyroxin.

Hawthorn and Motherwort (Crataegus laevigata *and* Leonurus cardiaca)

Both these herbs are heart tonics, helping to moderate heart rate. Hawthorn is considered the best cardiotonic in the world, and it is often effective in combating the heart palpitations that can be a symptom of hyperthyroidism. Motherwort has similar tonic effects and is especially good for heart conditions that are associated with anxiety and tension. This herb is also used as a tonic for the female reproductive system, making it a good choice for the female cat (or other female critter) suffering from hyperthyrodism.

Note that using either of these herbs may decrease the dosage of cardiac drugs needed to control heart palpitations, and extra caution should be used when cardiac beta-blockers have been prescribed. Always check with your veterinarian before starting any herbal therapy!

Plants for Hyper- and Hypothyroidism

Siberian ginseng *(Eleutherococcus senticosus)* helps prevent both thyroid atrophy and hyperplasia. Its adaptogenic qualities act to strengthen and balance all organ systems.

Licorice *(Glycyrrhiza glabra)* is another herb used for its adaptogenic qualities; it strengthens and balances the whole body. Licorice root is also a specific herb for the adrenal glands.

A Few Words about Hypothyroidism

Interestingly, although hypothyroidism is rare in cats, its most common cause is iatrogenic — destruction of the thyroid gland as a result of treatment for hyperthyroidism. So it is relatively easy to connect the common symptoms to the treatment being given. Typical symptoms of hypothyroidism include dry and scaly skin, lethargy, avoidance of cold areas, and weight gain.

The Allopathic Approach

Conventional treatment for hypothyroidism includes supplementing the cat's diet with one of several synthetic thyroxins; the idea is to come up with the dosage of the drug that resupplies the amount of the hormone that a normally functioning gland would provide. The problem with this approach is that because a supply of synthetic thyroid is readily available, the gland's feedback system tells it that it does not need to produce any more hormone. So the thyroid shuts down, and it may never again be able to function properly.

The Herbal Approach: Seaweeds

There are many types of seaweed herbs, the names of which are often used interchangeably, including:
- Bladderwrack (*Fucus vesiculosus*)
- Kelp (*Laminaria* spp.); often other species of seaweeds are simply called "kelp"
- Irish moss (*Chondrus crispus*)
- Nori (*Porphyra* spp.)
- Dulse (*Palmaria palmata*)
- Wakame (*Undaria* spp.)
- Kombu (*Laminaria* spp.)
- Arame (*Ecklonia bicyclis*)

All of these sea herbs contain high levels of vitamins and minerals, and they are the highest sources of plant iodine found anywhere. They are considered specific herbs for the underactive thyroid gland.

Other Herbs

When treating hypothyroidism, I try to think in terms of which organ systems seem to be the most adversely affected. For example, if the skin is showing severe signs of the disease, I would add skin-helper herbs, such as yellow dock, Oregon grape root, sarsaparilla, burdock, and/or licorice root. And since the liver is almost always involved in any disease process, I usually include a liver-specific herb, such as milk thistle or dandelion root.

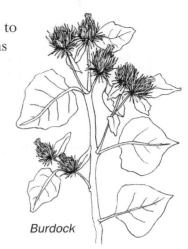

Burdock

CONSUMER ALERT

Heavy metals, especially mercury, can be toxic to the thyroid. Many of our vaccines are preserved with thimerosal, a combination of ethyl mercuric chloride, thiosalicylic acid, sodium hydroxide, and ethanol. (Vaccines may also contain a further litany of bad-guy stuff, including antibiotics, aluminum gels, formaldehyde, monosodium glutamate, egg proteins, and sulfites — each of which has been implicated in immune reactions in some individuals.)

According to a recently published warning from the ever-alert U.S. government, some human vaccines containing thimerosal, when given to infants, may produce internal levels of mercury that exceed recommended safety levels. Now, I don't know of any similar studies on thimerosal in animals, but I do know that many of our critter vaccines also contain it as a preservative. And I know that a half-pound kitten is a whole lot smaller than the normal-sized kid who is getting vaccinated.

Thimerosal: one more good reason to question the practice of annual vaccines for your cat.

The Urinary System

In veterinary lingo we call it UTI (urinary tract infection) or FUS (feline urological syndrome). To further confuse clients, we veterinarians sometimes add the sobriquet of feline urolithiasis, meaning "stones in the urinary tract." But for the average person, it is simply a "plugged" cat. The "plugged" tomcat is a relatively common condition, but it can be a persistently pesky problem to solve. Nevertheless, I've found that this disease responds to herbs better than to anything else I'd tried previously.

WHAT CAUSES THE PROBLEM?

Basically, a thick mucus-like substance that sometimes contains small, gravelly stones develops in the diseased cat's bladder and urethra (the bladder's outflow tube). We don't really know why some cats develop this substance; veterinary scientists have not discovered any one cause, although they have suspected and examined several, including nutrition and viral and bacterial infection.

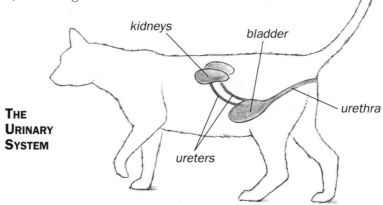

kidneys

bladder

urethra

THE
URINARY
SYSTEM

ureters

Especially in tomcats, the substance may completely plug the urethra. Then, as the bladder fills up, the cat has a life-threatening emergency condition that requires catheterization under anesthesia and considerable aftercare. Once plugged, a high percentage (50 to 75 percent) of these cats will have the same problem time and again, and often surgery is required to maintain urine flow. The surgery, called perineal urethrostomy, enlarges the urethra.

If used early enough, herbs can be helpful in preventing the worst of the FUS/UTI problems, and I use them routinely to help prevent recurrence of the syndrome as well as for other urinary diseases.

Symptoms of UTI/FUS

A plugged cat will often exhibit these symptoms:

- Frequent attempts to urinate; the cat is constantly scratching in and around the litter box
- Small amounts of urine (wet spots in the litter box are small)
- Straining; the cat spends lots of nonproductive time hunched over in the litter box
- Painful urination; the cat may cry whenever he eliminates
- Blood in urine; you may sometime see blood in the urine spots, but sometimes the blood can be seen only with a microscope
- Inappropriate urination; the cat urinates in unusual places, such as on the floor, the couch, or your pillow

First, take your cat to the veterinarian right away. The vet will want to do a urinalysis, and perhaps take X rays, do a CBC, or perform other tests. Important findings from the urinalysis include specific gravity (which measures the functional ability of the kidney tubules), pH (which may indicate infections or stones), and the presence of blood (indicating loss of integrity to the wall of the bladder, urethra, ureters, or kidneys), white blood cells (an indication of infection), or crystals (indicating the possibility of bladder stones). The urinalysis and other tests will help determine a diagnosis and will help in choosing the best treatment.

Treating with Herbs

With herbal therapy, we are trying to accomplish three major goals:

1. Increase urine flow. With this flushing action we help eliminate the bacteria that cause ongoing infections, and we can prevent recurrence of infections. Because chronic bladder infections are a cause of stone formation, by diluting the urine we are also decreasing the formation of stones. And, with a little luck, the increased urine flow may flush out smaller stones that have already formed.

2. Directly address any bladder infections. Some herbs have mild antibiotic activity, and many herbs help the animal's immune system deal with the invading organisms.

3. Coat the bladder and urethra with soothing herbs (urinary demulcents). Bladder irritation can cause a nerve reaction that ultimately leads to spastic contractions of the urethral walls, resulting in pooling of the urine and, thus, a better environment for infection and stone formation.

Dandelion (Taraxacum officinale)

The root of this herb is a potent diuretic, meaning that it will make your cat urinate frequently — provided he is not totally plugged. So, whenever you use dandelion, be absolutely certain that your cat's litter box attempts are productive. Otherwise you could merely be filling up the bladder quicker, which of course makes the condition worse, faster.

The theory behind using dandelion root is that a free flow of urine cleanses the urinary system, and the increased "go-ability," by itself, often clears up urinary diseases. But in addition to its diuretic action, dandelion provides specific healing actions for the liver and gallbladder and is also a wonderful general tonic. Since I believe that the bladder is often merely a repository for an animal's more general problems of the body, mind, and spirit, this is all the more reason for a general body tonic.

Dandelion

Incidentally, diuretics tend to cause a loss of potassium in the urine, and cats can be very sensitive to decreased levels of this important mineral. However, dandelion is an excellent source of potassium, naturally resupplying the loss.

Oregon Grape (Mahonia *spp.*)

Because we now recognize that goldenseal is a seriously threatened species, I have substituted Oregon grape root for the endangered herb — and I find it to be equally effective clinically. Oregon grape root's usefulness is due to its high levels of berberine, a substance with strong antimicrobial qualities. Because of the berberine, Oregon grape's primary use is for infections. In addition, the herb stimulates the flow of bile and, like dandelion, has general tonic properties.

If you can find an herbal product that contains a commercially grown source of organic goldenseal, you can substitute it for the Oregon grape root recommended here. However, another advantage of Oregon grape root is that it is relatively palatable; many cats hate the taste of goldenseal with a passion.

How to Use Dandelion and Oregon Grape

My best successes with these two herbs occur when we have caught the disease process in its very earliest stages; this makes observation all-important. I recommend small oral doses of 1 to 3 drops of the (nonalcoholic, if possible) tincture of each herb, 5 to 6 times a day. Continue until your cat returns to the normal number of trips to the litter box, has a normal flow (without straining), and produces good-sized puddles. At this point, cut back from this therapeutic dose to a preventive/maintenance dose. If your cat shows signs of a recurrence of active infection, return to the therapeutic dose.

For prevention or maintenance, use only the long-term tonic dandelion root. Give your cat one dose (several drops) of the tincture or sprinkle up to a teaspoon of the ground root on his food a few days each week. Long-term use of Oregon grape root (or any of the berberine-containing herbs) may decrease the normal, good-guy bacteria in the gut. Whenever you use Oregon grape root, add a teaspoonful or so of unsweetened yogurt to your cat's dinner dish.

Other Herbs

There are a couple of other herbs I consider using for urinary problems, depending on the specific condition.

Nettle. Otherwise known as stinging nettle, this herb is a diuretic, astringent, and general tonic that seems to be most useful for the animal that is experiencing painful urination. Nettle is also specific for respiratory allergies, and the root was recently proven effective for benign prostatic enlargement (BPE); add it to the herbal formula of any pet experiencing these symptoms. Dried nettle leaves do not sting like the fresh leaves, and they can be used long term as a general tonic, sprinkled on your cat's food. The leaves or roots can also be made into a tea to moisten the food.

Cranberry. Cranberry acidifies the urine, which helps control bacteria, and it contains a substance that acts as a barrier to keep bacteria from attaching to the bladder wall. All this is great for bacterial infections, but the problem is getting your cat to drink something that tastes of cranberry.

Cranberry capsules are an answer for easy-to-pill critters, but most herbal capsules are large, so they're not practical for cats. You can, of course, break open the capsules and hide the contents in your cat's food, but I have not had much luck with this method. However, there are exceptions to every rule, so don't let this deter you from trying cranberry on your cat. Remember, too, that most of the store-bought cranberry juices are sweetened and not appropriate for use; the sweetener will only make the urinary problem worse.

What to Do for Bloody Urine

Bloody urine is *not* something to fool around with; consult your vet immediately for an accurate diagnosis. After the vet has made a diagnosis and you are confident that you are on the right track therapeutically, there are some herbs that act as astringents — which tighten connective tissue, helping to control bleeding — or demulcents, which soothe irritated tissue and help prevent spastic contraction of the urethra.

The following herbs can be used to help your other therapies:
- **Astringents:** Horsetail *(Equisetum arvense)* and plantain *(Plantago* spp.)
- **Demulcents:** Corn silk *(Zea mays)* and marsh mallow leaf *(Althaea officinalis)*

part 3

The Herbal Repertory

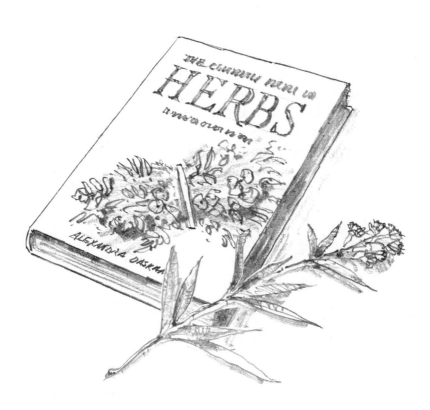

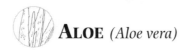 ALOE *(Aloe vera)*

Chemical Composition

A popular healing plant, aloe contains aloins, anthraquinones, and flavonoids.

Key Uses

The whole leaves and fresh or dehydrated juice from aloe are used mainly as a vulnerary (wound healer). This herb is an external demulcent and emollient (softening and soothing to the skin).

Current Research and Modern Uses

Internally, aloe is used when a strong cathartic (laxative with strong evacuant action) is indicated. Small doses act as an emmenagogue, increasing menstrual flow in human females.

Externally, the juice is used for burns, sunburn, wounds, insect bites, and so forth. It is one of the most effective healing agents for burns and injuries. Aloe relieves irritation as it heals.

Studies show that aloe has antibacterial and antifungal activity against a number of organisms, especially skin pathogens. It has proven activity against several viruses, including HIV-1. (Aloe reduces the amount of AZT required by as much as 90 percent.) Aloe has been approved, in injectable form, for veterinary use against fibrosarcomas and feline leukemia. The herb also enhances the function of the immune system and has anti-inflammatory and antiallergy activity.

Precautions and Side Effects

When aloe is taken internally, its laxative and cathartic effects can be dramatic. Since it stimulates uterine contractions, it should not be used internally during pregnancy. Aloe is also passed through the mother's milk, possibly exerting purgative effects on nursing animals.

Comments

I use aloe only externally; internal use has too much potential for adverse side effects. Aloe cannot be beaten as an external wound healer, especially for burns and superficial scrapes. I've found that some animals object to its application — possibly because of its astringent-like effects.

BLADDERWRACK *(Fucus vesiculosus)*

Chemical Composition

There are many species of seaweed or sea kelp (including hijiki, arame, kombu, and nori), and they are often used interchangeably with bladderwrack. Rich in algin, mannitol, carotene, and zeaxanthin, bladderwrack also contains polysaccharides, polyphenols, volatile oils, and other minerals, especially calcium.

Key Uses

The dried thallus or the whole plant is used as an antihypothyroid and a thyroid tonic. But it's also antirheumatic/antiarthritic, nutritive, and anti-inflammatory, and it stimulates metabolism.

Current Research and Modern Uses

Bladderwrack is used primarily for diseases of the thyroid, but it is also used to treat obesity, arteriosclerosis, and digestive disorders. For inflamed joints, it may be used both internally and externally (as a poultice). This seaweed provides building blocks needed by endocrine glands, making it helpful for endocrine imbalances. This is especially true in conditions affecting the female reproductive system.

Bladderwrack is an excellent food source and a wonderful supplement to the diet. It is rich in iodine. Recent work indicates that it may strengthen the immune system and, by this action, fight or prevent cancer.

Precautions and Side Effects

Allergic reactions have been known to occur with bladderwrack. Although the presence of too much iodine in the diet is said to possibly induce or worsen hyperthyroidism, you'd need to give your pet 33 pounds of seaweed daily to reach toxic levels.

Comments

In my practice, bladderwrack is a mainstay for hypothyroidism and many other glandular problems. I also think it's excellent for stimulating metabolism and reducing inflammation. Despite its fishy odor, not all animals enjoy the taste; camouflage it in food for a few days until your pet gets used to the flavor.

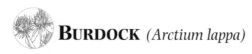

BURDOCK *(Arctium lappa)*

Chemical Composition

Burdock contains flavonoid glycosides, bitter glycosides, alkaloids, high amounts of inulin, vitamin
B_2, thiamin, iron, and silicon.

Key Uses

The roots, rhizomes, and seeds of burdock are used medicinally. The Chinese call the roots gobo. This herb is an alterative, diuretic,
and diaphoretic that is also nutritive. In addition, burdock is antioxidant
and antimicrobial.

Current Research and Modern Uses

Burdock root is a blood purifier; it's included in many formulas for toxin
elimination and bowel and lymphatic cleansing. It is often used to treat
arthritis and rheumatism. When taken as a tea or tincture, the root is
especially good for treating dry or scaly skin conditions, all forms of
eczema, and skin ailments related to arthritis.

Burdock promotes kidney function and cleans the liver. Recent studies
indicate that burdock has antibacterial and antifungal activity, possibly as
a function of its antioxidant biochemicals. One of its major constituents,
inulin, is anti-inflammatory and helps correct imbalances of the immune
system. Some evidence indicates antitumor activity in burdock, an action
that may be enhanced if burdock is combined with red clover.

Precautions and Side Effects

Rare cases of contact dermatitis from the leaves have been reported.
Internally, burdock has no known serious side effects, though diarrhea
may occur with extended use.

Comments

For its blood-cleansing capabilities and alterative powers, I add burdock
to most of my herbal prescriptions — especially for arthritis, skin problems of all kinds, and toxin-related conditions (particularly toxic or
chronic bowel syndrome). Use the chopped roots as a sprinkle or a tincture (for the finicky eater).

CALENDULA *(Calendula officinalis)*

Chemical Composition

The active constituents in calendula are saponins, carotenoids, bitter principles, essential oils, sterols, flavonoids, mucilage, and tocopherols. The fresh plant contains salicylic acid, which acts as an analgesic.

Key Uses

The flowers of calendula, which is often called pot marigold (not to be confused with the ornamental marigolds, *Tagetes* spp., that are commonly grown in flower gardens), help to stimulate wound healing. This herb is also a good astringent, liver-function enhancer, febrifuge (fever reducer), and tonic herb.

Current Research and Modern Uses

Many studies indicate that calendula flowers are antimicrobial, antifungal, antibacterial, antiviral, and vulnerary. They also stimulate the immune system, inhibit some tumors, have a calming effect on the nervous system, and aid liver function.

Externally, calendula is used for all types of wounds — cuts, scrapes, abrasions, burns, and inflammations of the mouth and pharynx. It is especially effective for wounds that heal poorly. Use it as a poultice on sprains and bruises.

Calendula promotes the reconstruction of tissue by enhancing fibroblastic growth; its anti-inflammatory activity decreases swelling and discharge as well as the scarring that normally occurs from burns, abscesses, and abrasions.

Precautions and Side Effects

Calendula is generally recognized to have no adverse side effects.

Comments

When made into a tea or ointment for use on open wounds, calendula is my favorite wound healer. It is so good, in fact, that I have to caution folks not to use it on wounds that need to drain (abscesses, for example), as they may heal over too quickly.

CATNIP *(Nepeta cataria)*

Chemical Composition

Catnip contains the essential oils cavracol, geraniol, citronellol, neroli, pulegone, nepetalic acid, thymol, and nepetalactone. It also has tannins, vitamins C and E, magnesium, manganese, and flavonoids.

Key Uses

In almost all animals, catnip acts as a sedative (in cats, the sedation is preceded by euphoric or aphrodisiac effects, a reaction not seen in dogs or other animals). It has nervine, carminative, antispasmodic, antipyretic, diaphoretic, and diuretic properties. The herb is also a stomachic (digestive tonic) and light emmenagogue, and it increases gallbladder activity.

Current Research and Modern Uses

The probable cause of a cat's blissful reaction to catnip is nepetalactone, a component of the essential oil that mimics a cat's sexual pheromones. Nepetalactone is also similar to the sedative constituents of valerian (see page 180), which may explain its sedative action in dogs and other animals.

Catnip has a mild tranquilizing effect on most animals, making it a good treatment for restlessness, nervousness, and insomnia. It is a gentle nervine that is also excellent for gastrointestinal upsets, such as colic, flatulence, diarrhea, and dyspepsia. Its diaphoretic activity makes it good for the early symptoms of colds, flus, and other feverish conditions, especially bronchitis.

Externally, catnip is used as an antiseptic poultice for sores and wounds. Dr. James Duke, a noted herbalist, has seen promising results using catnip to help prevent and slow the progression of cataracts.

Precautions and Side Effects

No significant side effects have been reported with catnip.

Comments

Catnip is a great calming herb for most cats. Simply toss a handful of the fresh herb near your cat and wait for the euphoria to subside. Use it intermittently on long trips to ease nervousness. Other animals are susceptible to catnip's calming effects, but without the initial euphoria seen in cats.

CAYENNE (*Capsicum* spp.)

Chemical Composition

The main constituents of cayenne are capsaicin; red coloring matter; and oleic, palmetic, and stearic acids. The herb is high in calcium, phosphorus, iron, and zinc as well as vitamins A, B, and C. (Its vitamin C content is greater per ounce than that of oranges, and it nearly doubles as the fruit ripens.)

Key Uses

Also known as chili pepper, the fresh and dried fruit of the cayenne plant is employed as a stimulant for all body systems. In addition, it has tonic, carminative, diaphoretic, rubefacient, hemostatic, and antioxidant properties.

Current Research and Modern Uses

Cayenne is an outstanding carrier herb that helps transport other herbs and medicines to various parts of the body, especially the heart, stomach, and brain. A useful systemic stimulant, cayenne regulates blood flow and strengthens the heart, arteries, capillaries, and nerves.

Cayenne is a general tonic that is also specific for the circulatory and digestive systems, and it balances blood pressure. In small amounts it aids digestion, stimulating the appetite and dispelling gas. It also eases the pains of arthritis and rheumatism and the itching of skin conditions. Cayenne can be used topically for those ailments as well.

In tests cayenne has been shown to slow the development of some cancers, possibly because of its high levels of vitamins and antioxidants.

Precautions and Side Effects

Very high doses of cayenne over long periods of time can cause problems, such as chronic gastritis, kidney and liver damage, and neurological effects. External applications may cause blistering.

Comments

Surprisingly, many pets have a hankering for spicy foods, making administration of cayenne easy. I find the herb especially helpful for treating arthritis pain, poor circulation, and heart conditions. I generally don't recommend topical applications, however.

CHAMOMILE (Roman, *Anthemus nobilis;* German, *Matricaria recutita*)

Chemical Composition

The volatile oil of chamomile contains chamazulene, isadol, mucilage, coumarin, and flavone glycosides.

Key Uses

Chamomile's flowers are an effective carminative, relieving gas and distention of the stomach. The plant is also anti-inflammatory, analgesic (pain relieving), and antiseptic. Its vulnerary action makes it an excellent topical wound healer.

Current Research and Modern Uses

Chamomile has a seemingly endless list of uses. Europeans have long used it to treat colic, diarrhea, insomnia, indigestion, toothache, swollen gums, skin problems, gout, sciatica, some cancers, and more. Perhaps the best indication of how Europeans feel about chamomile is the German saying *alles zutraut* — "capable of anything."

A gentle sedative that is safe for even young animals, chamomile can be used to alleviate anxiety, insomnia, and indigestion. Animal tests indicate that chamomile causes a reduction of aggressive behavior.

In addition to being effective against some bacteria and fungi, chamomile has anti-inflammatory activity that makes it ideal for inflamed eyes, sore throats, and other irritations. It is an excellent choice for gas, flatulence, and sore tummies, as well.

Precautions and Side Effects

No serious side effects or drug interactions are known. As with any herb, there is a small potential for sensitization.

Comments

Chamomile is my favorite sedative — one cup of tea, and I'm snoring in my favorite chair. It seems to work equally well with some pets. I like to add chamomile to topical treatments (in tea-spritzer, ointment, or oil-based forms) because I think it calms the irritable animal while healing the wound.

DANDELION *(Taraxacum officinale)*

Chemical Composition

Dandelion contains taraxacin (a crystalline bitter), taraxacerin (an acrid resin), and inulin. The roots and leaves contain variable amounts of vitamins A, C, E, and B complex; potassium (up to 5 percent); calcium; iron; thiamin; choline; lecithin; and riboflavin. The leaves have more beta-carotene than carrots do.

Key Uses

As a diuretic, dandelion stimulates the urinary organs. It's a tonic and general stimulant, especially for the urinary system and liver. The herb is also supportive of the liver and gallbladder, and it's used to treat gallstones.

Current Research and Modern Uses

In animal studies, dandelion has proved to be a strong diuretic, with an action comparable to that of the drug furosemide. But while furosemide depletes potassium from the body, dandelion resupplies it naturally.

Dandelion is one of the strongest cholagogues, increasing the liver's production of bile by more than 50 percent. In addition, the plant is a choleretic; it increases bile flow to the gallbladder. This benefits patients with colitis, liver congestion, gallstones, and several forms of liver insufficiency.

Precautions and Side Effects

There are virtually no reported side effects, but topical contact with the sap of the stems may produce allergic reactions in sensitive people. Since dandelion is a diuretic, remember to keep the litter box clean and fresh

Comments

In treating urinary disorders, I have had more luck using dandelion root than anything else for tomcats with feline urological syndrome (FUS), I've found dandelion in combination with Oregon grape root, to be unparalleled.

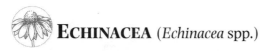

ECHINACEA (*Echinacea* spp.)

Chemical Composition

The *Echinacea* genus has an assortment of active constituents that can be divided into seven categories: polysaccharides, flavonoids, caffeic acid derivatives, essential oils, polyacetylenes, alkylamides, and miscellaneous chemicals. Amounts of the chemicals vary between leaf and root preparations, among different species, and at different times of the year.

Key Uses

Echinacea is the best choice to balance the immune system and is effective against all types of infections.

Current Research and Modern Uses

There is a vast amount of pharmacological information on echinacea. Studies have indicated that the herb elevates white blood cell count when it is low (but not when it is normal or high), promotes nonspecific T-lymphocyte activation, and enhances macrophage phagocytosis. It also has a mild, direct effect against bacteria, viruses, and yeasts. Most of the antimicrobial activity is probably due to its effects on the immune system.

Echinacea also promotes tissue regeneration and reduces inflammation. It possesses indirect anticancer activity via its general immuno-enhancing effects. In addition, echinacea has anti-inflammatory activity that helps alleviate rheumatoid arthritis.

Precautions and Side Effects

Echinacea is not toxic when used at recommended doses. In fact, chronic administration of the plant to rats at doses many times the human therapeutic dose produced no evidence of toxic effects. Mutagenic tests with echinacea demonstrated no cancer-causing activity.

Comments

I would not (and could not) practice holistic medicine without echinacea. In today's world I see mostly chronic diseases — arthritis, cancers, reactions to drugs — that I feel are immune-system related. Many of these conditions respond well to echinacea.

EYEBRIGHT (*Euphrasia officinalis*)

Chemical Composition

The main constituents of eyebright are glycosides (including aucubin), phenolic acid, tannins, resins, and volatile oil.

Key Uses

An astringent and anti-inflammatory, eyebright is also used as an anticatarrhal and expectorant.

Current Research and Modern Uses

Eyebright's best-known use is for conditions of the eye — particularly chronic inflammation, stinging and weeping eyes, and eyes that are overly sensitive to light. However, the herb can be used for treating infections of the mucous membranes, including sinusitis and nasal congestion.

Eyebright is effective when used internally as a tea or tincture, or externally as an eyewash.

Precautions and Side Effects

No serious adverse reactions have been reported.

Comments

Eyebright is simply the best medicine available for the red, irritated eye. I even use my animal eyewashes on myself! If I think an eye is infected, I usually add another antibiotic herb, such as elder, goldenrod, or goldenseal, to the mixture. For all eye infections, I like to use eyebright internally in combination with other antibiotic and toxin-cleansing herbs, such as echinacea, Oregon grape root, and possibly burdock root or cleavers.

GINGER *(Zingiber officinale)*

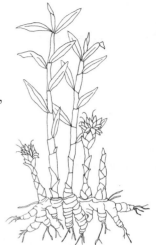

Chemical Composition

At least 477 chemicals — including essential oils, gingerols, shogaols, and phenolic compounds — have been isolated in ginger. Because the bio-chemicals are present in different concentrations in the fresh and dried plant, choose a combination of the two for the best effect.

Key Uses

The root of this Asian plant is used as a stimulant to revive and enhance the function of many organ systems. It's also an antispasmodic and carminative, and it can be applied topically as a rube-facient (to increase blood flow and heat in the treated region). As a diaphoretic, ginger increases circulation and sweating.

Current Research and Modern Uses

Ginger is an excellent herb for debilitated animals — particularly those with poor appetites; poor circulation and cold limbs; a deep, slow pulse; and general pallor. The herb's antispasmodic activity works to ease coughs, nausea, and pains of the stomach and lower back. It also helps alleviate all sorts of digestive problems, including diarrhea, colic, and flatulence.

Externally, ginger can be used as a poultice to treat muscle pains and strains and fibrositis. Ginger is mildly tonic to all organ systems.

Precautions and Side Effects

Because of its great warming ability, ginger should be used with caution in temperamental animals. The herb should be used in moderation during pregnancy.

Comments

Ginger is a wonder herb that's good for lots of ailments. But many animals don't like its taste, at least not initially. Animals that have been exposed to ginger's unique flavor during healthy periods appreciate it more on the days when they don't feel well.

GINKGO *(Ginkgo biloba)*

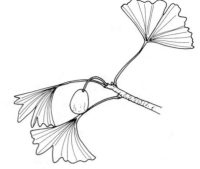

Chemical Composition

This herb contains terpine lactones (or ginkgoglides) and flavone glycosides (flavonoids).

Key Uses

Ginkgo acts on two major systems of the body: the nervous and cardiovascular systems. Almost every medical condition that ginkgo successfully treats is due, at least in part, to poor circulation.

Current Research and Modern Uses

Dozens of human studies and hundreds of animal studies have confirmed ginkgo's medicinal effects. It enhances vitality by increasing blood flow to the brain, strengthening brain cells by acting as a free-radical scavenger, and making the transmission of nerve messages more effective. It is helpful in treating Alzheimer's disease, dementia (dimming mind syndrome), and depression. This herb enhances both long-term and short-term memory in youngsters and the elderly alike.

Ginkgo improves circulation by preventing or reducing the release of platelet-activating factor (PAF), the substance that increases stickiness. Ginkgo also helps maintain the integrity and elasticity of the blood vessels and reduces the tendency of vessels to contract and constrict (vasospasm) during times of stress.

Precautions and Side Effects

Ginkgo acts as a blood thinner; patients who are taking blood-thinning drugs (including aspirin) should not use ginkgo without first consulting a doctor or herbalist.

Rare side effects — including nausea, headache, dizziness, excessive bruising or bleeding from minor cuts, and bloodshot eyes — have been reported. (Interestingly, most patients note relief from headaches and dizziness while on ginkgo.) No particular adverse side effects have been found with long-term use. Patients often require several months of ginkgo use before results become noticeable.

GINSENG

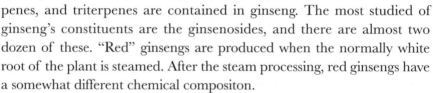

(Asian, Panax ginseng; American, Panax quinquefolius; Siberian, Eleutherococcus senticosus)

Chemical Composition

Saponins, sugars, lipids, vitamins, minerals, proteins, phenolic compounds (salicylic acid), terpenes, and triterpenes are contained in ginseng. The most studied of ginseng's constituents are the ginsenosides, and there are almost two dozen of these. "Red" ginsengs are produced when the normally white root of the plant is steamed. After the steam processing, red ginsengs have a somewhat different chemical compositon.

Key Uses

Ginseng is an adaptogenic and stimulant. This whole-body tonic is an especially good cardiac stimulant.

Current Research and Modern Uses

Panax ginseng is considered the king of tonics — it supplies energy to the entire body, helping it recover from stress, fatigue, weakness, and deficiencies. It is reported to have the power to move people to their physical peak, increasing vitality as well as physical performance and mental acuity. The ginsengs function as adaptogens; they restore normality and increase nonspecific resistance to disease or other changes. Siberian ginseng was the original herb that was referred to as an adaptogen.

Comments

Ginseng is excellent for many ailments, but I do not prescribe it often for several reasons. First, it's very difficult to know what you're getting when you buy ginseng. Several studies have analyzed ginseng products from Asia, and many of these products did not contain the amounts of the herb stated on the label; some contained none. Second, there are several species of ginseng, and each has a slightly different medicinal activity; customers are often confused by the varieties. Third, our indigenous ginseng, *Panax quinquefolium,* is threatened by overharvesting in the wild. Finally, ginseng is hard to grow, and it takes several years for the rootstock to develop its full medicinal potential.

GOLDENSEAL *(Hydrastis canadensis)*

Chemical Composition

All parts of goldenseal, but especially the rhizome, contain several alkaloids: hydrastine, berberine, and canadine.

Key Uses

Goldenseal has many uses, mainly acting as an alterative, anti-inflammatory, astringent, antibiotic, antifungal, and cholagogue. It also has laxative, muscular stimulant, oxytocic (uterine stimulant), antitumor, and hemostatic properties.

Current Research and Modern Uses

Good for any inflammatory condition, goldenseal is especially helpful for inflammation of the mucous membranes (gastrointestinal, upper respiratory, urinary, reproductive, eye, mouth, throat, and sinus). This herb fights bacterial, viral, and fungal infections and can be used as an external wash for inflammation or infection of the eyes.

Use goldenseal for digestive problems and liver conditions. Goldenseal is valuable for treating loss of appetite, skin wounds or chronic skin conditions, infectious diarrhea, fevers, and lymph cleansing.

Precautions and Side Effects

Do not use goldenseal during pregnancy. The herb may alter blood pressure, and prolonged use (more than 2 weeks) alters the gut flora. High doses of goldenseal may interfere with vitamin-B metabolism, and the fresh plant can cause inflammation of mucous tissue in sensitive animals. In addition, some animals really dislike its taste.

Comments

Goldenseal is a wonder herb, but it is at risk of becoming an endangered species. If you can find a reliable source of organically grown goldenseal, by all means, use it. But if the label says "wildcrafted," please use Oregon grape root, an effective alternative.

HAWTHORN *(Crataegus laevigata)*

Chemical Composition

Hawthorn's major constituents are saponins, glyco-sides, flavonoids, acids (including ascorbic acid), and tannins. The berries also contain cardiotonic amines, choline and acetylcholine, and purine derivatives.

Key Uses

The ripe fruit of hawthorn is used as a cardiac tonic and hypotensive (to relax peripheral blood vessels). This herb is also astringent and diuretic.

Current Research and Modern Uses

Hawthorn is perhaps the world's best cardiotonic. It improves metabolic processes in the myocardium (which enhances the general function of the heart), dilates coronary blood vessels (thus improving coronary blood supply), and abolishes some types of rhythm disturbances. Hawthorn normalizes heart activity, either depressing or stimulating it, depending on the need. It is a good herb for heart failure or weakness.

Hawthorn is safer and milder in activity than digitalis, a popular med-ication. There are no cumulative effects with this herb (as with digitalis), and hawthorn may correct the undesirable side effects of that drug. The herb even has a synergistic effect with the medication; dosages of both can be reduced by about half when they are used in combination.

Hawthorn acts to stabilize collagen, resulting in decreased capillary permeability and fragility. In addition, the berries also strengthen appetite and digestion and are a good remedy for nervousness and insomnia.

Precautions and Side Effects

Health risks or adverse side effects from hawthorn have not been recorded. Since hawthorn potentiates the action of digitalis, consult an herbalist before taking hawthorn with it or any other cardiac drug.

Comments

If a patient has cardiac problems of any type, I recommend hawthorn. It is slow and gentle in its action, but it does not have adverse side effects.

KAVA KAVA *(Piper methysticum)*

Chemical Composition

The active ingredients of kava kava, found in the fat-soluble portion of the root and rhizome, include kava lactones or kava pyrones.

Key Uses

The rhizomes of kava kava, whose botanical name means "intoxicating pepper," are used to relieve anxiety and conditions related to tension and restlessness.

Current Research and Modern Uses

Kava kava, a plant native to the Pacific islands, relaxes the central nervous system without affecting mental sharpness; users actually exhibit improved memory and reaction time. Your pet won't build up a tolerance to the plant, so you won't need to keep increasing the dosage.

Studies have shown that kava kava creates changes in EEG patterns that are typical of antianxiety drugs — but without their sedative effects. It influences the brain's limbic system; researchers suspect that this action contributes to kava kava's muscle-relaxant and pain-reducing effects. The herb is a more potent analgesic than aspirin.

Kava kava can also be used to induce sleep. It is not a sedative but, rather, a hypnotic: It calms the mind and allows it to drift off, without any hangover the next morning. Used topically, kava kava acts as a local anesthetic, with effects comparable to those of the drug procaine. This plant is also effective against fungal skin infections.

Precautions and Side Effects

Kava kava can create mild gastrointestinal disturbances. Long-term or excessive use may cause a yellowing or rash of the skin or equilibrium problems. Consult an herbalist before using kava kava with barbiturates, antidepressants, or other drugs that act on the central nervous system. Do not use kava kava during pregnancy.

Comments

I use kava kava to help animals relax. I've found it especially helpful to calm nervous animals before athletic competitions or chiropractic adjustments.

LICORICE *(Glycyrrhiza glabra)*

Chemical Composition

The root of this plant contains glycosides (mainly glycyrrhizin), saponins, flavonoids, bitter principles, volatile oil, coumarins, asparagine, and estrogenic substances.

Key Uses

An adrenal-supporting herb, licorice is also used to soothe irritated membranes — especially those in the gastrointestinal tract (such as ulcers). This plant is an anti-inflammatory, antimicrobial, antiarthritic, tonic, and adaptogen (enhances the body's ability to adapt). It's often used to treat the liver and respiratory problems, such as bronchitis and coughs.

Current Research and Modern Uses

Glycyrrhizin, one of the plant's major active constituents, has a chemical structure similar to that of natural corticosteroids. Thus, licorice stimulates the secretion of hormones by the adrenal glands. The herb is an anti-inflammatory, reducing joint swelling and easing some skin conditions. Licorice raises the concentration of prostaglandins in the digestive system, promoting new cell growth and alleviating ulcers. It soothes irritated membranes and relieves abdominal colic by promoting mucus secretion in the stomach. It also prolongs stomach-cell life and decreases the secretion of pepsin.

Licorice root, which has antitussive, demulcent, and expectorant qualities, has long been used to alleviate coughs. It compares favorably to codeine in experiments. Research has also proved licorice root effective in treating liver toxicity. When the whole root (rather than an extract) is used, licorice acts as a tonic.

Precautions and Side Effects

Reported side effects include sodium retention and potassium loss, resulting in edema (accumulation of fluids within tissues); hypertension (high blood pressure); and hypokalemia (abnormally low potassium in the blood). Do not use licorice for patients with heart or liver disease or for patients who tend to retain sodium.

MILK THISTLE *(Silybum marianum)*

Chemical Composition

An important herb for liver ailments, milk thistle contains flavolignans (primarily silymarin, as well as silybin, silydianin, and silychristin), essential oils, bitter principles, and mucilage.

Key Uses

Milk thistle is the best available treatment for the liver. It also promotes milk secretion in the lactating female.

Current Research and Modern Uses

Few plant principles have been as extensively researched in recent years as milk thistle's primary active ingredient, silymarin. This chemical helps stabilize liver cell membranes and stimulates protein synthesis while also accelerating cell regeneration in liver tissue cells that are damaged by alcohol, drugs, and chronic liver disease.

Double-blind studies have shown milk thistle to be supportive in treating chronic inflammatory liver disorders, such as hepatitis, cirrhosis, and fatty infiltration of the liver. In addition, silymarin is considered a specific antidote for poisoning from the amanita (deathcap) mushroom. A few European studies even suggest that silymarin may help treat the scaly skin patches of psoriasis. Milk thistle is so safe that it can be used even by breast-feeding mothers.

Precautions and Side Effects

Rare mild laxative effects have been reported.

Comments

Milk thistle is without question the best therapy I have found for all sorts of liver conditions. Western medicine just does not have anything comparable. In addition to using it for specific liver maladies, I often add milk thistle to my herbal prescriptions because no matter what the disease, the liver is active in detoxification and metabolism.

MOTHERWORT *(Leonurus cardiaca)*

Chemical Composition

Motherwort is composed of bitter glycosides (including leonurin and leonuridine), alkaloids (including leonuinine and stachydrene), volatile oil, and tannins.

Key Uses

Motherwort's aerial parts, which are gathered at flowering, have cardiac tonic properties. The herb is also known for promoting menstruation and acting as a sedative and antispasmodic.

Current Research and Modern Uses

Motherwort is primarily used as as a support for the female reproductive system and as a cardiac tonic to strengthen the heart without straining it. While motherwort is a specific herb for an overrapid heart rate, it is also good for most heart conditions, especially those associated with anxiety and tension. Motherwort is much like valerian — it is hypotensive and sedative.

Motherwort is not really a uterine tonic; rather, it works more as a uterine stimulant. This herb is used during the first stages of pregnancy to prepare the uterus for childbirth and in the later stages of pregnancy to ease childbirth and promote contractions. It is also a useful tonic for menopausal changes.

Precautions and Side Effects

No serious side effects have been reported. Sensitive patients may develop contact dermatitis from exposure to the leaves or flowers.

Comments

For heart problems I think of hawthorn first; then I consider motherwort. I think some patients can use its added sedative effects. I recommend motherwort for some of my spayed female patients with heart conditions, because spaying creates a condition similar to that which occurs in human women at menopause.

I do occasionally take motherwort myself, hoping for a part, if not all, of the 300-year life span enjoyed by a Chinese sage who drank motherwort tea every day.

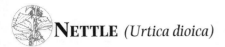

NETTLE *(Urtica dioica)*

Chemical Composition

Nettle contains indoles, including histamine and serotonin; formic acid; chlorophyll; glucoquinine; iron; vitamins A, C, and K; acetylcholine; silicon; protein; and fiber.

Key Uses

Also known as stinging nettle, the leaves of this herb are nutritive, supplying important vitamins and minerals to the whole body. Its tonic effects are well known among herbalists. Nettle is also a diuretic, galactagogue (enhancing milk production), hemostatic, and astringent.

Current Research and Modern Uses

As a general tonic, nettle strengthens, supports, and provides nutrients to the whole body. Because of its high iron content, it is beneficial for treating anemia.

The root offers good antibiotic possibilities; its high sterol levels enhance the production of white blood cells. A poultice of the astringent leaves may be used for nosebleeds or other hemorrhagic conditions, such as uterine bleeding.

This herb has been used for a variety of urinary complaints, including urinary stones, nephritis, cystitis, and the swelling of benign prostatic hyperplasia (BPH). Other conditions that have been successfully treated with nettle include eczema and other skin conditions, arthritis, rheumatism, stomach problems, and lung ailments, such as asthma.

Precautions and Side Effects

No serious side effects are known, but a few rare allergic reactions have been observed. Unless handled carefully with gloved hands, the fresh leaves — which have sharp, barblike projections — can cause a stinging sensation. Cooked and dried leaves lose this property.

Comments

One of my favorite nutritive herbs, nettle is a great general tonic. It makes a tasty tea and sprinkle that most animals take when it is added to their food.

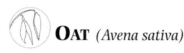 OAT *(Avena sativa)*

Chemical Composition

The active ingredients of oat are soluble oligosaccharides and polysaccharides, salicylic acid, steroid saponins, amino acids, magnesium, calcium, and flavonoids.

Key Uses

The fresh or dried aboveground parts of oats are most frequently employed, but other parts are also used: the milky, still-green fruits; the ripe, dried fruits; and the dried leaf and stem. Oat makes an excellent nervine tonic, and it even has antidepressant properties. Oat is also nutritive, demulcent, and vulnerary.

Current Research and Modern Uses

Oat is one of the best remedies for feeding the nervous system (either alone or in combination with other nervines), especially when it is under stress. The herb is used as a tonic to balance the mind, body, and spirit. Oat is considered a specific in cases of nervous debility and exhaustion associated with depression, as well as for general debility. Recently, this herb has been used as a sexual tonic for both males and females.

Externally, oat makes a wonderfully soothing remedy for skin conditions. Several oat bath products for animals are commercially available, but you can easily make your own. Boil about 1 pound of shredded, organic oat straw in 2 quarts of water for about ½ hour. Strain the liquid and add it to your pet's bathwater, just before the final rinse.

Precautions and Side Effects

No health problems have been associated with oat.

Comments

I add oat to almost all my herbal prescriptions because most sick animals are anxious about their conditions. The herb is also readily accepted by most animals, especially in the form of oatmeal.

OREGON GRAPE (*Mahonia* spp.)

Chemical Composition

A good source of berberine and several other alkaloids (including hydrastine), Oregon grape also contains resins and tannins.

Key Uses

This plant has strong antibiotic and skin-healing effects. It stimulates bile production, has immune-stimulating activity, and lowers fevers. *Note:* At the present time, most herbalists substitute Oregon grape root for goldenseal, which is being wild-harvested to the point of near extinction. The two herbs have similar components, and Oregon grape root may actually be better for skin conditions.

Current Research and Modern Uses

Oregon grape root is used to treat infections and inflammations that affect the mucous membranes of the respiratory, digestive, and genitourinary tracts. Berberine, a major constituent of the plant, has broad-spectrum activity against bacteria, protozoans, fungi, and yeasts. It also inhibits adherence of Group A streptococcal bacteria to host cells.

Oregon grape root stimulates the immune system by activating macrophages and increasing blood supply to the spleen. In human and rat studies, Oregon grape root demonstrated an activity against brain tumors (by stimulating white blood cells) that is stronger than that of the currently used chemotherapy agents.

Precautions and Side Effects

Oregon grape root is generally nontoxic at recommended dosages. Do not use it during pregnancy, however. High doses may interfere with the metabolism of B vitamins.

Comments

Oregon grape root might not be quite as strong as antibiotic drugs, but since berberine is effective against yeast, I see none of the bothersome yeast overgrowths that occur with antibiotic use. For prolonged periods, I recommend the addition of natural "good-guy" bugs, such as lactobacilli, supplied in yogurt or in supplement form.

RED CLOVER *(Trifolium pratense)*

Chemical Composition

Red clover contains phenolic glycosides, flavonoids, coumarin derivatives, cyanogenic glycosides, vitamins and minerals, and volatile oils (methyl salicylate and others). The herb also has isoflavones, which possess estrogen-like activity.

Key Uses

The blossoms of red clover are used as an alterative, expectorant, and antispasmodic. They also promote skin healing and may have antitumor activity.

Current Research and Modern Uses

As an alterative, red clover is used to treat a wide range of skin conditions, such as eczema, eruptions, and psoriasis. An expectorant, red clover is helpful for treating coughs and bronchitis. It has a mild, relaxing nervine quality and can be used along with or in place of chamomile.

Red clover is what herbalists refer to as a blood purifier, which means it helps remove accumulated toxins. Research suggests that the herb may have anticancer effects in animals, perhaps because of its high levels of carotene and vitamin E. Most herbalists, when treating cancers of various types, combine red clover with other suitable herbs.

Precautions and Side Effects

No side effects are known when the herb is used at recommended doses. Because of its high coumarin levels (coumarin inhibits blood clotting) and estrogenic-like compounds, I am cautious when using red clover in pregnant patients or those with bleeding disorders.

Comments

Red clover is another one of those herbs that is "good for what ails you," and it's readily accepted by most animals either as a tea or food sprinkle. I almost always combine red clover with burdock root because the two seem to act synergistically. All my cancer patients take red clover in combination with other appropriate herbs.

SARSAPARILLA (*Smilax* spp.)

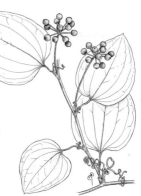

Chemical Composition

Sarsaparilla is recognized for its steroid saponins, including sarsaponin, smilasaponin, and sarsaparilloside; and its aglycones, including sarsasapogenin, smilagenin, and pollinastanol. The herb also contains starch, resins, and a trace of volatile oil.

Key Uses

The roots and rhizomes of sarsaparilla are anti-inflammatory, making the herb particularly good for skin diseases. It also has antiarthritic properties, which may stem from the anti-inflammatory effects. As a diaphoretic and antipyretic, sarsaparilla causes sweating and lowers fevers. It's also a diuretic, alterative, and tonic, enhancing the balance of all body systems.

Current Research and Modern Uses

Sarsaparilla is used most often for chronic diseases, such as arthritis and skin conditions. It is especially good for scaly skin conditions, including psoriasis and eczema, in which there is a lot of irritation.

The saponins in sarsaparilla bind bacterial toxins in the gut — this is possibly due to its activity as a blood purifier, alterative, and antipyretic. The herb has been used as a male reproductive-system stimulant, but this use is questionable. While it contains chemicals that can be converted to testosterone in a test tube, it's doubtful that conversion can occur in the body.

Precautions and Side Effects

No serious side effects are known to have occurred with the use of sarsaparilla, but stomach upset and kidney irritation may occur in rare cases.

Comments

I try to include sarsaparilla, which is readily accepted by most animals, in all herbal prescriptions for skin ailments and chronic arthritic conditions. Because it is an alterative and blood cleanser, it's good in combination with such herbs as burdock and yellow dock.

SLIPPERY ELM *(Ulmus rubra)*

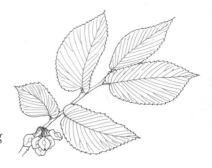

Chemical Composition

With mucilage similar to that in mucilage-rich linseed, slippery elm coats, soothes, protects, and rejuvenates areas suffering from infection, inflammation, and other irritants.

Key Uses

Slippery elm soothes irritated mucous membranes and eases diarrhea. It's also used internally for stomach ulcers, colitis, sore throats, and coughs and topically for wounds and abscesses.

Current Research and Modern Uses

Native Americans used slippery elm bark for dysentery, diarrhea, and ulcers. They also used a topical poultice of the herb to treat sores and wounds. The USDA currently lists slippery elm bark as a safe and effective demulcent (a substance that provides a protective coating and soothes irritated tissues) that can be taken orally.

Precautions and Side Effects

Prolonged use (more than 3 weeks) in high dosages may overcoat the intestinal tract and prevent absorption of nutrients.

Comments

Slippery elm is absolutely the best remedy I've come across for the animal with a nervous stomach. No one traveling with a pet should be without it. The show animal who frets before a performance will almost certainly benefit from a dose of slippery elm. I also use this herb in combination with other modalities, such as homeopathy and acupuncture, when treating more severe cases of intestinal upset — colitis, ulcerative colitis, ulcers, and so on.

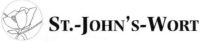

ST.-JOHN'S-WORT
(Hypericum perforatum)

Chemical Composition

St.-John's-wort contains numerous compounds with documented biological activity, the naphthodi-anthrones hypericin and pseudohypericin, a broad range of flavonoids, essential oils, and xanthones.

Key Uses

This popular antidepressant is also an antiviral. When used topically and in oral tinctures, St.-John's-wort has wound-healing capabilities.

Current Research and Modern Uses

St.-John's-wort is one of the most scientifically studied and most used herbs (especially in Germany) in today's herbal pharmacopeia. At least two dozen randomized trials conducted on several thousand humans with mild to moderately severe depressive disorders have shown responses to St.-John's-wort that are as good as or better than those seen with currently available pharmaceutical antidepressives.

Two of the plant's constituents, hypericin and pseudohypericin, inhibit a variety of encapsulated viruses, including herpes simplex type 1 and 2, human HIV-1, murine cytomegalovirus, and parainfluenza-3 virus. In addition, hypericin prevents tumor cell growth and induces tumor cell death by inhibiting protein kinase C. An excellent wound healer, hypericin extracts appear to have an antibacterial action against gram-positive organisms and also increase new cell formation.

Precautions and Side Effects

St.-John's-wort extract seems to be relatively free of side effects. The most frequently noted side effects are gastrointestinal irritation, allergic reaction, fatigue, and restlessness. St.-John's-wort is known to cause photosensitization (and occasionally loss of appetite, nervousness, coma, and possibly death) in cattle, horses, rabbits, sheep, and swine. I have not found reports of photosensitization in cats, but I always advise clients who have light-skinned cats to keep them out of bright sunlight while their pets are using St.-John's-wort.

TURMERIC *(Curcuma longa)*

Chemical Composition

Turmeric is a member of the ginger family, and it contains a mix of phenolics called curcumin. Other active ingredients include volatile oil (with tumerone and zingiberene), cineole and other monoterpenes, sugars, starch, protein, and high amounts of vitamin A and other vitamins and minerals.

Key Uses

The rhizome of turmeric is used as both an antioxidant and anti-inflammatory. It's a good choice for liver conditions, irritable bowel syndrome, and other gastrointestinal problems. Turmeric is an antimicrobial and anticarcinogen that is used for cardiovascular ailments.

Current Research and Modern Uses

Turmeric has liver-protecting properties: It stimulates the flow of bile (increasing output by as much as 100 percent) and increases its solubility.

Tests indicate that the anti-inflammatory effects of turmeric are comparable to those of cortisone and phenylbutazone. In addition, turmeric has long been used as a carminative for decreasing gas formation; reducing intestinal spasms; and increasing secretion of secretin, gastrin, bicarbonate, and pancreatic enzymes.

The positive cardiovascular effects of turmeric include lowered cholesterol levels, inhibited platelet aggregation, interference with intestinal cholesterol uptake, increased conversion of cholesterol into bile acids, and increased excretion of bile acids.

Turmeric has potential as an anticancer herb. It interferes in all steps of cancer formation: initiation, promotion, and progression.

Precautions and Side Effects

No toxicity has been reported at normal intake levels. With very high amounts, inflammation or ulceration of the stomach lining may occur.

Comments

While most culinary herbs have medicinal value, turmeric has potent therapeutic activities against a wide variety of ailments. It's also easy to dose for most pets; simply sprinkle some over their food.

VALERIAN *(Valeriana officinalis)*

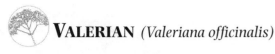

Chemical Composition

Another famous herb, valerian contains volatile oils (valepotriates, valerianic acid, valeranone, and valernal), esters, and alkaloids.

Key Uses

Valerian is used as a nervine tonic to calm nervous disorders from tension, anxiety, and discomfort. It's an antispasmodic, sedative, and pain reliever that is also good for upset stomachs.

Current Research and Modern Uses

Recent studies have shown that this herb sedates and regulates the autonomic nervous system and relieves tension and restlessness. When used in animals, valerian typically decreases unrest, anxiety, and aggressiveness without decreasing reaction time. Oddly, reaction time is actually improved with valerian.

A primary sedative for sleep disorders associated with anxiety, nervousness, exhaustion, headache, and hysteria, valerian acts as a tranquilizer that calms nervous-system imbalances, both physical and psychological. Many studies confirm the herb's usefulness for insomnia, but not all cases of insomnia respond to valerian. The herb is rapidly metabolized; the effects are gone by morning, leaving no side effects or morning "hangover."

Precautions and Side Effects

The whole root (rather than an extract) of valerian is virtually without toxicity. Approximately 5 percent of people respond to valerian with hyperactivity. If this occurs in your pet, simply discontinue use.

Comments

I find valerian very effective for most animals with separation anxiety or insomnia — the nighttime pacer, whiner, and crier. I like to use it both before and after surgery or during any prolonged disease, the times when Pet is the most anxious.

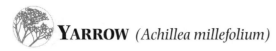

YARROW *(Achillea millefolium)*

Chemical Composition

Yarrow's active ingredients include volatile oils, sesquiterpene lactones, alkamids, flavones, and a bitter substance called achilleine.

Key Uses

The flowers and leaves of yarrow are used to stop blood flow. The plant is also used for loss of appetite; for liver, gallbladder, and stomach complaints; and as an antipyretic. In addition, yarrow is antiseptic, anti-inflammatory, analgesic, and diaphoretic. The flowers are thought to have more potent medicinal qualities than the leaves.

Current Research and Modern Uses

The common name soldier's wound wort is a key to yarrow's primary external use — to stop the bleeding and infection of "battle wounds," such as cuts, scrapes, and abrasions. A poultice of the flowers and leaves stems blood flow from a fresh wound, as long as it is not bleeding profusely.

Internally, yarrow is used to aid the liver, soothe upset stomachs, and improve poor digestion. It is probably one of the best herbs for lowering fevers. Traditionally, yarrow has also been used to treat inflammatory conditions of the joints.

Precautions and Side Effects

Yarrow may cause contact dermatitis. It can also cause photosensitization and other allergic reactions.

Comments

I've mostly used yarrow as an external wound dressing. In my part of the country, yarrow grows wild in most of the pasturelands that are riddled with rocks and flint outcroppings. Thus, the herb is readily available when we (and our rambunctious grandkids) fall and are most likely to need it.

Some of my holistic veterinary friends have used yarrow internally more than I have, and many of them have found it to be an excellent herb for fevers, colds, and flulike symptoms.

YELLOW DOCK *(Rumex crispus)*

Chemical Composition

Yellow dock's primary chemical constituents are anthro-quinone glycosides, tannins, and oxalic acid. It is also high in iron, vitamins, and thiamine.

Key Uses

Used to treat dry, itchy skin, yellow dock is also a blood cleanser.

Current Research and Modern Uses

Yellow dock is typically used as an alterative (blood cleanser), but investigations into this use haven't uncovered any one cause for its successful clinical applications. The herb's thiamine content is one suspected reason. Yellow dock also has mild antibacterial activities.

Of all the herbs, yellow dock has one of the strongest reputations for clearing up skin problems, liver and gallbladder ailments (Native Americans used it to treat jaundice), and glandular inflammation and swelling. Its high iron content makes it an effective treatment for anemia. Conditions that respond well to yellow dock include eczema, ringworm, psoriasis, and cancer.

Precautions and Side Effects

No side effects have been reported at recommended doses. The oxalic acid in yellow dock's leaves and roots, if taken in large doses, may be irritating to the intestinal tract.

Comments

In my practice I recommend yellow dock — often in combination with other herbs, such as licorice root and Oregon grape root — for all skin-related problems. I also use yellow dock whenever I think blood cleansing would benefit the patient. Most of my patients with chronic conditions benefit from a general detox formula that includes yellow dock.

Other Useful Herbs

ARTICHOKE *(Cynara scolymus)*

The fresh or dried leaves of artichoke are used as a liver tonic and protective, with damage-preventing properties similar to those of milk thistle. This popular food stimulates the regeneration of liver cells and is also a bitter. It protects the body from toxins, restores healthy growth of liver cells, increases the amount of bile available for digestion, and reduces blood cholesterol and other fats. And it's generally recognized as safe with no known toxicity. If your pet doesn't like the taste of milk thistle or turmeric, artichoke is a good alternative.

BLACK COHOSH *(Cimicifuga racemosa)*

The dried roots and rhizomes of black cohosh contain resin, bitter glycosides, ranunculin, salicylic acid, tannin, and phytoestrogens. Black cohosh's primary use is as a normalizer and relaxant for the female reproductive tract. It may also be used for arthritic and rheumatic pains and to reduce spasms associated with coughs. For reproductive problems it combines well with blue cohosh. No health hazards are known to exist with proper use.

Most often I use black cohosh in combination with other reproductive herbs — dong quai, blue cohosh, wild yam, vitex, motherwort, and secondary herbs — as well as acupuncture and other alternative methods. I have been pleased with black cohosh's results for a variety of female problems.

BUGLEWEED *(Lycopus virginicus, L. europaeus)*

The aerial parts of bugleweed are specific for the overactive thyroid; they inhibit the peripheral deiodination of the thyroid hormone thyroxin. This herb will also aid a weak heart when there is an associated buildup of water in the body, and it acts as a sedative for cough relief, especially when the cough is of a nervous nature.

DONG QUAI *(Angelica sinensis)*

Dong quai is also known as Chinese angelica; the roots and rhizomes of this plant are used as a uterine tonic, antispasmodic, and alterative. Sometimes called the "female ginseng," dong quai is used in human medicine to treat almost all female gynecological ailments, especially menstrual cramps, irregularity, it delayed flow, and weakness. It is also a good herb to relieve the symptoms of menopause. In general, dong quai is an excellent tonic for the reproductive tract. In addition, it is an antispas-modic for insomnia, hypertension, and cramps. It is nourishing to the blood, making it a useful blood purifier and treatment for anemia.

Dong quai can cause photosensitivity. Do not use the herb during pregnancy or for patients with diabetes.

IRISH MOSS *(Chondrus crispus)*

Like bladderwrack, Irish moss is a seaweed. The dried thallus contains carrageenins, iodine, bromine, iron, other mineral salts, vitamins A and B_1, and up to 80 percent mucilage. This herb is an expectorant and demulcent used mainly for respiratory problems such as bronchitis. It is also used for digestive conditions such as gastritis and ulcers, and it has been applied topically to sores and ulcers. The carrageenin in Irish moss is used as a binding agent in the food industry to make jellies, aspic, and other products, and in the cosmetics industry as a skin softener.

Irish moss is commonly prepared as syrup in combination with Iceland moss *(Cetraria islandica)* and blackstrap molasses.

MULLEIN *(Verbascum thapsus)*

The leaves, flowers, and occasionally the roots are used as a demulcent, anodyne, antispasmodic, astringent, mild diuretic, expectorant, nonnar-cotic analgesic, mild sedative, and vulnerary. This plant is most useful for treating ailments of the lungs, such as coughs, sore throat, and bronchitis; ears, particularly infections; urinary tract, including infections and incon-tinence; stomach, especially cramps and intestinal catarrh; and nervous system, to induce sleep and relieve pain and headaches. Although the fine hairs on the leaves and flowers of mullein can be irritating to some, this problem is eliminated by straining the tea or tincture before use.

PARSLEY *(Petroselinum crispum)*

Parsley is a breath freshener, diuretic, and mild laxative that has hypoten-sive and antimicrobial properties. It has also been used to treat liver prob-lems and gallstones. Its estrogenic qualities help promote menstruation and milk production. Parsley is a good herb to use after meals to prevent bad breath. However, make sure that Pet does not have any underlying conditions, such as dental problems or digestive upsets, that may be caus-ing halitosis.

Do not use parsley during pregnancy. The herb may cause nerve inflammation if used to excess.

SAW PALMETTO *(Serenoa repens)*

This herb's primary effects are on the digestive tract, stimulating the appetite and increasing body weight. It also has calming qualities that are good for Pet's general health and disposition. Saw palmetto is frequently used to tone and strengthen the male reproductive system and as a treatment for benign prostatic hyperplasia (BHP) and infections of the prostate and urogenital organs.

No side effects have been reported when saw palmetto is used as recommended. Stomach complaints, though rare, may occur.

THYME *(Thymus spp.)*

Thyme has expectorant, antispasmodic, antimicrobial, astringent, and carminative qualities. It is a good remedy for coughs, asthma, and chronic or acute bronchitis, and also treats dyspepsia and sluggish digestion. When used externally, its strong antiseptic properties help heal wounds.

Because thyme is a uterine stimulant, it should not be used during pregnancy. Skin sensitivity is also a possibility when it is used externally.

WALNUT *(Juglans spp.)*

Walnut has astringent and anthelmintic properties. In Europe, the herb is a popular remedy for skin and eye conditions. I use walnut flower essence quite often for animals undergoing transitions, such as a move to a new home, the loss of a companion, the addition of a new member to the family, or any form of physical or emotional change.

The herb may cause digestive disorders with prolonged use.

YUCCA *(Yucca spp.)*

Although yucca is used to treat liver and gallbladder disorders, arthritis, hip dyspasia, and joint injuries, research substantiating its efficacy has not been conclusive. I occasionally employ yucca for short-term use in cases of arthritis. However, I have not been impressed with the consistency of the results. While I have never seen any problems with yucca, I am cautious to watch for intestinal complaints.

Yucca can be purgative and cause intestinal cramping. Long-term use may slow the absorption of fat-soluble vitamins.

Glossary

Adaptogen. A nontoxic agent that increases an organism's ability to adapt. Adaptogenic herbs work well with other herbs (and other medicines), generally adding to their activities.

Alterative. Acts as a blood purifier, gradually restoring the body to its proper state of health and vitality. Alteratives are used to treat toxicity of the blood, infections, arthritis, cancer, and skin eruptions. Alteratives also help the body assimilate nutrients and eliminate the waste products of metabolism.

Analgesic. Able to reduce pain.

Anthelmintic. Able to destroy or expel worms from the digestive tract.

Antiabortive. Helps inhibit the termination of a pregnancy.

Antiasthmatic. Relieves symptoms of asthma by dilating bronchioles or breaking up mucus.

Antibiotic. Inhibits the growth of or destroys microorganisms, including bacteria, viruses, protozoans, and fungi. While herbal antibiotics often have direct germ-killing effects, many of them also stimulate the body's own immune response.

Anticatarrhal. Helps the body remove excess mucus buildup, whether in the sinuses or in other parts of the body.

Antiemetic. Reduces nausea to relieve or prevent vomiting.

Antifungal. Inhibits fungal infestations.

Anti-inflammatory. Inhibits inflammation.

Antilithic. *See* **Lithotriptics.**

Antipyretic. Reduces or prevents fevers.

Antirheumatic. An agent used for the symptomatic treatment of rheumatism.

Antiseptic. An agent applied to the skin to prevent the growth of microorganisms.

Antispasmodic. Prevents or relaxes muscle spasms or cramps.

Antitussive. Prevents or inhibits coughs.

Antiviral. Inhibits viral infections.

Aphrodisiac. Increases sexual potency, appetite, or sensitivity.

Aromatic. Having a strong and often pleasant odor that can stimulate the digestive system. Aromatics are often used to add aroma and taste to other medicinals.

Astringent. An agent with a constricting or binding effect. Astringents are commonly used to stop hemorrhages, discharges, and secretions and to treat swollen tissues.

Bitter. A bitter-tasting herb that acts as a stimulant for the digestive system through the taste buds.

Cardiotonic. Increases heart tone and function.

Carminative. Relieves intestinal gas and severe pains of the bowels. Carminatives are rich in volatile oils, which stimulate peristalsis of the digestive system and relax the stomach.

Cathartic or laxative. Clears the bowels.

Cholagogue. Promotes the flow of bile into the small intestine. Cholagogues also have a laxative effect, since bile is our internally produced, all-natural laxative.

Demulcent. Soothes irritated membranes, especially mucous membranes.

Diaphoretic. Induces sweating, thus aiding the skin in the elimination of toxins.

Diuretic. Increases the secretion and elimination of urine. Diuretics help eliminate internal toxins and treat water retention, lymph swellings, infections of the urinary tract, skin conditions, and stones and gravel of the urinary system.

Emetic. Induces vomiting and causes the stomach to empty.

Emmenagogue. Promotes or regulates menstruation, stimulating and normalizing menstrual flow. Emmenagogues also act as tonics to the female reproductive system.

Emollients. When applied to the skin, emollients soften, soothe, or protect.

Expectorant. Expels mucus from the lungs and throat.

Febrifuge. *See* **Antipyretic.**

Galactogogue. Increases the flow of milk in a nursing female.

Hemostatic. Arrests hemorrhaging.

Hepatic. Tones and strengthens the liver and increases the flow of bile. *See also* **Cholagogue.**

Hypnotic. Induces sleep without inducing a hypnotic trance.

Laxative. *See* **Cathartic.**

Lithotriptic. Helps dissolve and eliminate urinary and biliary stones and gravel.

Mucilage. Gelatinous constituents of herbs that act as demulcents and emollients.

Nervine. Tones and strengthens the nervous system. Some nervines act as stimulants; some act as relaxants.

Oxytocic. Stimulates contraction of the uterus.

Parasiticide. *See* **Anthelmintic.**

Pectoral. Strengthens and heals the respiratory system.

Purgative. *See* **Cathartic.**

Rubefacient. When applied to the skin, rubrifacients cause a gentle local irritation and stimulation and dilation of the capillaries, thus increasing circulation to the region. Rubrifacients draw inflammation and congestion from deeper areas, making them useful for the treatment of sprains, arthritis, rheumatism, and other problems involving the joints.

Sedative. Calms the nervous system and reduces stress and nervousness throughout the body.

Sialagogue. Stimulates the flow of saliva, aiding in the digestion of starches.

Soporific. Sleep-producing herbs. *See also* **Hypnotics.**

Stimulant. Increases the activity of a specific organ system or the whole body.

Styptic. Stops external bleeding through astringency. *See also* **Astringent.**

Tonic. Strengthens and enlivens specific organs or the whole body. Most tonics have general effects on the whole body, but they also typically have a marked effect on a specific organ system.

Vulnerary. When applied externally, vulneraries aid in the healing of wounds and cuts by promoting cell growth and repair.

Organ System Tonic Herbs

ORGAN SYSTEM	TONIC HERBS
Immune system	Astragalus, echinacea, ginseng (all species), licorice, schisandra
Nervous system	Chamomile, ginkgo, Siberian ginseng, hop, lemon balm, lobelia, passionflower, peppermint, skullcap, valerian
Cardiovascular system	Bugleweed, cayenne, Siberian ginseng, hawthorn, kelp, motherwort, rosemary, turmeric, valerian
Musculoskeletal system	Alfalfa, devil's claw, echinacea, horsetail, licorice, sarsaparilla, saw palmetto, wild yam, yarrow
Liver and biliary	Dandelion, goldenseal, Oregon grape, parsley, rhubarb, sassafras, wild yam
Digestive system	Artichoke, dandelion, gentian, ginger, milk thistle, turmeric
Female reproductive system	Black cohosh, black haw, cramp bark, chaste tree, dong quai, ginger, licorice, red raspberry, valerian
Male reproductive system	Burdock, damiana, Siberian ginseng, licorice, pumpkin seed, pygeum, sarsaparilla, saw palmetto

Herbs for Specific Conditions

Before you begin using a remedy listed here, be sure that you read all about the herb in part 3. Also, consult the chapters on specific conditions for more information.

CONDITION	INTERNAL HERBS	EXTERNAL HERBS
Abscess	Cayenne, cleavers, echinacea, garlic, goldenseal, marsh mallow root, oregano	Calendula, chamomile, comfrey, lavender, marsh mallow root, plantain, St.-John's-wort, yarrow
Acne	Burdock root, cleavers, dandelion root, echinacea, licorice root, red clover, sarsaparilla	
Allergic rhinitis (see Upper respiratory disease)		
Allergies	Astragalus, dandelion root, echinacea, fenugreek, goldenseal, licorice root, milk thistle, nettle, Oregon grape root, thyme, turmeric	
Anxiety	Catnip, chamomile, hop, kava kava, lavender, oat, passionflower, St.-John's-wort, skullcap, valerian	
Arrhythmia (see Cardiovascular disease)		
Arthritis	Antiarthritics: alfalfa, devil's claw, frankincense, turmeric, yucca; For pain and inflammation: cayenne, feverfew, licorice root, St.-John's-wort, willow bark, wild yam; Antioxidants: basil, celery seed, ginger, oregano, parsley, thyme	
Asthma	Astragalus, ginkgo, licorice, mullein	
Bacterial or viral infection	Calendula, cat's claw, chaparral, echinacea, elder, garlic, ginger, goldenseal, lavender, licorice root, myrrh, oregano, Oregon grape root, Pau d'arco, rose, rosemary, St.-John's-wort, thyme, yarrow	
Bad breath	Dill, fennel, parsley	

CONDITION	INTERNAL HERBS	EXTERNAL HERBS
Bladder infection (see Urinary tract infection)		
Bladder stones (see Urinary tract infection)		
Blepharitis (see Conjunctivitis)		
Bronchitis	Astragalus, coltsfoot, echinacea, goldenseal, licorice root, marsh mallow, mullein, Oregon grape root, osha root, plantain, thyme	
Burns		Aloe (for pain, add a pinch of echinacea and/or kava kava) or make a poultice of one or more of the following: calendula, chamomile, comfrey, plantain, St.-John's-wort)
Cardiovascular disease	Heart specifics: hawthorn, motherwort; Diuretics: dandelion root; Heart supporters: cayenne, ginger, ginkgo, *Panax ginseng;* Nervines: oat	
Cataracts	Bilberry, eyebright; Antioxidants: basil, celery seed, ginger, oregano, parsley, thyme	Eyebright
Circulatory problems	Cayenne, ginger, ginkgo	
Cognitive dysfunction (dimming mind syndrome)	Ginkgo, Siberian ginseng	
Colic	Aniseed, caraway, cardamom, catnip, cayenne, chamomile, cinnamon, coriander, dill, fennel, ginger, licorice root, peppermint, valerian	
Colitis	Chamomile, licorice root, marsh mallow, peppermint, slippery elm	
Conjunctivitis	Bilberry, echinacea, eyebright, goldenseal, Oregon grape root	Calendula, chamomile, eyebright
Constipation	Aloe, cascara sagrada, flaxseed, licorice root, senna, slippery elm, yellow dock	

CONDITION	INTERNAL HERBS	EXTERNAL HERBS
Cough	Coltsfoot, licorice root, mullein, osha root, plantain, red sage, thyme	
Cuts and scrapes		Aloe, calendula, chamomile, chickweed, cleavers, comfrey, elder, garlic, goldenseal, lavender, mullein, myrrh, plantain, red sage, self-heal, St.-John's-wort, yarrow
Cystitis (see Urinary tract infection)		
Diarrhea	Goldenseal, licorice root, Oregon grape root, slippery elm	
Digestive problems (see Indigestion)		
Ear infection	Echinacea, goldenseal, oregano, Oregon grape root, thyme	Calendula, chamomile, clove oil, mullein, St.-John's-wort, witch hazel
Eczema and other inflammatory skin disorders	Burdock root, chickweed, cleavers, echinacea, goldenseal, nettle, Oregon grape root, red clover, sarsaparilla, yellow dock	Calendula, comfrey, lavender, nettle, yarrow
Epilepsy (see Seizures)		
Fever	Diaphoretics: catnip, cayenne, elder, ginger, peppermint, thyme, yarrow (*Note:* Since most fevers accompany an infection, see also Bacterial or viral infection)	
Flatulence (see Gas)		
Fungal infection		Arborvitae, calendula, echinacea, garlic, goldenseal
Gas	Aniseed, caraway, cardamom, catnip, cayenne, chamomile, cinnamon, clove, coriander, fennel, ginger, parsley, peppermint, thyme, valerian	
Gastritis	Chamomile, goldenseal, licorice, marsh mallow, slippery elm	

CONDITION	INTERNAL HERBS	EXTERNAL HERBS
Hepatitis	Artichoke, dandelion root, milk thistle, turmeric (*Note:* Also include herbs for bacterial infection)	
Hyperthyroidism	Bugleweed; Herbs for the heart: hawthorn, motherwart	
Hypothyroidism	Licorice, seaweed, Siberian ginseng	
Impotence	Damiana, ginkgo, *Panax ginseng,* saw palmetto	
Incontinence (see also Urinary tract infection)	Agrimony, horsetail	
Indigestion (dyspepsia)	Cardamom, catnip, cayenne, chamomile, cinnamon, clove, dandelion root, dill, fennel, ginger, peppermint, red sage, rosemary, thyme, valerian, wild yam	
Infection	Cayenne, cleavers, echinacea, garlic, ginger, goldenseal, lavender, myrrh, Oregon grape root, thyme	Echinacea, garlic, goldenseal, lavender, myrrh, Oregon grape root, thyme
Irritable bowel syndrome (see Colitis)		
Itching	Burdock root, calendula, chamomile, chickweed, cleavers, goldenseal, licorice root, Oregon grape root, sarsaparilla, St.-John's-wort, wild yam	Calendula, chamomile, echinacea, goldenseal, lavender, mullein, Oregon grape root, St.-John's-wort
Jaundice (see Hepatitis)		
Kidney disease	Cranberry (unsweetened juice), dandelion root, goldenseal, horsetail, marsh mallow root, Oregon grape root, parsley, Siberian ginseng, uva-ursi	
Kidney stones (see Urinary tract infection)		
Liver disease (see Hepatitis)		
Lyme disease and other tickborne diseases	Cat's claw, garlic, goldenseal, oregano, Oregon grape root	
Motion sickness	Ginger	

CONDITION	INTERNAL HERBS	EXTERNAL HERBS
Muscle sprains, strains, and pain	Arnica (homeopathic remedy only), cayenne, kava kava, licorice root, St.-John's-wort, turmeric, wild yam, willow bark	Arnica
Nephritis (see Kidney disease)		
Osteoarthritis (see Arthritis)		
Pain (general)	Black cohosh, black willow, cayenne, chamomile, hop, Jamaican dogwood, kava kava, licorice root, rosemary, St.-John's-wort, skullcap, turmeric, valerian, wild lettuce, wild yam	Arnica, chamomile, echinacea, mullein
Pancreatitis	Dandelion root, goldenseal, licorice root, slippery elm	
Pink eye (see Conjunctivitis)		
Prostate disorders	Damiana, goldenseal, horsetail, nettle, oregano, Oregon grape root, pygeum, saw palmetto	
Psoriasis	Burdock, cleavers, flaxseed, licorice root, milk thistle, Oregon grape root, red clover, sarsaparilla, yellow dock	
Rheumatism (see Arthritis)		
Ringworm (see Fungal infection)		
Seizures	Chamomile, ginkgo, kava kava, licorice root, milk thistle, passionflower, skullcap, St.-John's-wort, valerian	
Sinusitis (see Upper respiratory disease)		
Stomach upset (see Indigestion)		
Ulcers	Goldenseal, licorice root, marsh mallow, Oregon grape root, slippery elm	
Ulcerative colitis (see Colitis)		

CONDITION	INTERNAL HERBS	EXTERNAL HERBS
Upper respiratory disease	Chamomile, echinacea, elder, eyebright, garlic, goldenseal, mullein, myrrh, oregano, Oregon grape root, peppermint, rose hip, thyme, yarrow	
Urinary tract infection	Cranberry (unsweetened juice), dandelion root, goldenseal, marsh mallow root, nettle, Oregon grape root, parsley, plantain, uva-ursi	
Viral infection (see Bacterial or viral infection)		
Vomiting	Cinnamon, clove, marsh mallow, meadowsweet, peppermint, rosemary, slippery elm	
Wart	Arborvitae (herbal and homeopathic)	Arborvitae (herbal and homeopathic), banana peel
Wounds (see Cuts and scrapes)		
Yeast infection (see Fungal infection)		

Resources

For information on holistic veterinarians in your area, contact the American Holistic Veterinary Medicine Association at the address below. The Association's Web site lists holistic veterinarians by state and specifies the types of alternative medicine that each vet uses.

American Holistic Veterinary Medicine Association
2218 Old Emmorton Road
Bel Air, MD 21015
410-569-0795
AHVMA@compuserve.com
www.altvetmed.com

SUGGESTED READING

General Holistic Health Care Books for Pets

Frazier, Anitra. *The New Natural Cat*. Dutton, 1990.
Levy, Juliette de Bairacli. *Cats Naturally*. Faber and Faber, 1991.
Levy, Juliette de Bairacli. *The Complete Herbal Handbook for the Dog and Cat*. Faber and Faber, 1995.
Pitcairn, Richard. *Dr. Pitcairn's Complete Guide to Natural Health for Dogs and Cats*. Rodale, 1995.

General Herbal Books

Buhner, Stephen Harrod. *Herbal Antibiotics*. Storey Books, 1999.
Duke, James A. *The Green Pharmacy*. Rodale, 1997.
Foster, Steven. *Herbal Renaissance*. Gibbs Smith, 1993.
Foster, Steven and Varro E. Tyler. *Tyler's Honest Herbal*. Hawthorn Herbal Press, 1999.

Gladstar, Rosemary. *Herbal Healing for Women*. Fireside, 1993.
Gladstar, Rosemary. *Rosemary Gladstar's Herbal Remedies for Children's Health*. Storey Books, 1999.
Hoffman, David. *The New Holistic Herbal*. Element, 1991.
Mowery, Daniel B. *Herbal Tonic Therapies*. Random House, 1996.
Murray, Michael. *The Healing Power of Herbs*. Prima Publishing, 1995.
Tierra, Michael. *Way of Herbs*. Pocket Books, 1998.
Wood, Matthew. *The Book of Herbal Wisdom*. North Atlantic Books, 1997.

Magazines

The Herb Companion
428 North Cleveland Avenue
Loveland, CO 80537-5655
www.discoverherbs.com
Subscriptions:
P.O. Box 7714
Red Oak, IA 51591-0714
800-456-5835

Herbalgram (The Journal of the American Botanical Council and Herb Research Foundation)
P.O. Box 144345
Austin, TX 78714-4345
512-926-4900
www.herbalgram.org
Subscriptions:
800-373-7105

Herbs for Health
201 East Fourth Street
Loveland, CO 80537-5655
www.discoverherbs.com
Subscriptions:
P.O. Box 7714
Red Oak, IA 51591-0714
800-456-6018

The Whole Dog Journal (an excellent holistic newsletter with occasional herbal information)
1175 Regent Street
Alameda, CA 94501
510-749-1080
After November 1, 2000, visit our Web sites for holistic veterinary information, herbal updates, and fun stuff:

www.HonoringTheAnimals.com
www.HookedOnHerbs.com

Index

Note: Page number in *italic* refer to illustrations; those in **boldface** refer to charts.

Other Storey Titles
You Will Enjoy

Dr. Kidd's Guide to Herbal Cat Care, by Randy Kidd, DVM. Ever wonder how to enhance your cat's health with herbs? This guide shows you how to treat and prevent diseases of 15 body systems with all-natural herbal medicine. 192 pages. Paperback. ISBN 1-58017-188-5.

The Guilt-Free Dog Owner's Guide, by Diana Delmar. If you're short on time and space, these easy-to-read chapters will remove the anxieties associated with selecting the right dog, housebreaking, exercise, manners, behavior problems, home hazards, travel, and more. 180 pages. Paperback. ISBN 0-88266-575-8.

Your Puppy, Your Dog, by Pat Storer. Both parents and children can use this thorough guide to choosing, feeding, grooming, exercising, and training a new puppy. 128 pages. Paperback. ISBN 0-88266-959-1.

Help! My Puppy Is Driving Me Crazy, by Diana Delmar. In a fun question-and-answer format, this book offers humane, commonsense solutions for chewing, barking, grooming, eating, house-training, and other puppy problems. 192 pages. Paperback. ISBN 0-88266-992-3.

50 Simple Ways to Pamper Your Dog, by Arden Moore. Want to show your dog just how much he means to you? Then try these no-fuss tips for playing with, grooming, socializing, and feeding your dog into health and happiness. 144 pages. Paperback. ISBN 1-58017-310-1.

50 Simple Ways to Pamper Your Cat, by Arden Moore. If your favorite feline could use a little indulging, look no further! This book offers all the grooming, socializing, feeding, and playing tips you'll need to make your cat feel like a king. 144 pages. Paperback. ISBN 1-58017-311-X.

Growing 101 Herbs That Heal, by Tammi Hartung. Complete instructions for growing 101 medicinal plants using totally organic techniques. Hartung shares the secrets of growing and harvesting, as well as herb-by-herb profiles and a guide to creating homemade medicines. 256 pages. Paperback. ISBN 1-58017-215-6.

The Herbal Home Remedy Book, by Joyce A. Wardwell. Learn how to use 25 popular herbs to make simple herbal remedies to relieve common illnesses and enhance general health and well-being. 176 pages. Paperback. ISBN 1-58017-016-1.

These books and other Storey books are available at your bookstore, farm store, garden center, or directly from Storey Books, Schoolhouse Road, Pownal, Vermont 05261, or by calling 1-800-441-5700. Or visit our Web site at www.storeybooks.com